Guided Care

Chad Boult, MD, MPH, MBA. Dr. Chad Boult is the Eugene and Mildred Lipitz Professor of Health Policy & Management at the Johns Hopkins Bloomberg School of Public Health. He directs the Roger C. Lipitz Center for Integrated Health Care and holds joint appointments on the faculties of the Johns Hopkins University Schools of Medicine and Nursing. A geriatrician for more than 20 years, he has extensive experience in developing, testing, evaluating, and diffusing new models of health care for older adults.

Jean Giddens, PhD, RN. Dr. Jean Giddens is a professor and Senior Associate Dean for Academic Affairs at the College of Nursing, University of New Mexico in Albuquerque. A nurse educator for 25 years, her expertise is curriculum development and online learning applications. She has been involved with Guided Care as a nursing consultant since 2005.

Katherine Frey, MPH. Katherine Frey is a research associate in the Department of Health Policy & Management at the Johns Hopkins Bloomberg School of Public Health. As a project director for 8 years, she has extensive experience coordinating and managing large research studies. She also has rich experience in planning and delivering training programs for educating professionals.

Lisa Reider, MHS. Lisa Reider is a research associate in the Department of Health Policy & Management at the Johns Hopkins Bloomberg School of Public Health. She has 5 years of experience coordinating aging-focused research studies at Johns Hopkins University, with expertise in managing and analyzing large data sets. She is the project director of the Guided Care study.

Tracy Novak, MHS. Tracy Novak is a research associate in the Department of Health Policy & Management at the Johns Hopkins Bloomberg School of Public Health. As a health policy professional, her experience focuses on developing and implementing diffusion strategies, and organizing grassroots advocacy campaigns to build effective lobbying platforms. She has been an advocate on end-of-life issues and has testified before the Maryland House of Delegates in support of advance directives legislation. Her current work involves communicating information about Guided Care to relevant stakeholders and supporting its adoption in the American health care system.

Guided Care

A New Nurse–Physician Partnership in Chronic Care

CHAD BOULT, MD, MPH, MBA
JEAN GIDDENS, PhD, RN
KATHERINE FREY, MPH
LISA REIDER, MHS
TRACY NOVAK, MHS

SPRINGER PUBLISHING COMPANY

New York

Springer Publishing Company, LLC
11 West 42nd Street
New York, NY 10036
www.springerpub.com

Acquisitions Editor: Allan Graubard
Production Editor: Julia Rosen
Cover Design: Steve Pisano
Composition: Apex CoVantage

10 11 / 5 4 3 2

Library of Congress Cataloging-in-Publication Data

Guided care : a new nurse-physician partnership in chronic care /
Chad Boult . . . [et al.].
    p. ; cm.
  Includes bibliographical references and index.
  ISBN 978–0–8261–4411–9 (alk. paper)
  1. Chronically ill—Care.   2. Geriatric nursing.   3. Geriatric health
care teams.   I. Boult, Chad.
    [DNLM: 1. Chronic Disease—nursing.   2. Nursing Care—
methods.   3. Physician-Nurse Relations.   WY 152 G946 2009]
  RC108.G85   2009
  616'.044—dc22   2008050930

Printed in the United States of America by Yurchak Printing.

*To the many brave patients who struggle
every day to cope with chronic illnesses
in the chaotic U.S. health care system*

Contents

Foreword

The quality of medical care for older Americans and the future of American primary care are tightly linked. The vast majority of multiproblem older patients receive their care in primary care, and will continue to do so for the foreseeable future. But primary care is in crisis with looming physician shortages, and burnt out, unhappy practitioners working harder and harder. The burnout is almost certainly linked to their progressively older and sicker practice populations, which have made the work of primary care more complicated and time-consuming. Primary care has been described as being on a hamster wheel running faster and faster just to keep up. As a result, primary care physician visits are more rushed, which makes it even more difficult to meet the needs of older patients. The future of primary care and the quality of care for older, sicker adults may well depend on finding approaches to improving the efficiency and effectiveness of their primary care.

Several different strategies have been tried to remedy this problem with only limited success to date. The most common has been nurse care management, whereby nurses outside the practice provide educational, supportive, and some clinical services to high-risk patients. In most of these interventions, the nurses have little or no face-to-face contact with patients or their medical care team, which may account for their minimal impact on patient health and function (Chen, Brown, Esposito, Schore, & Shapiro, 2008). Three other tested interventions have attempted to locate nurses and other geriatric providers in primary care practices. Our group tested an intervention that had a geriatrician and geriatric nurse practitioner regularly see patients in primary care practices and make recommendations to the primary care team. We found no evidence of improvements in health or health care utilization such as reduced hospital visits (Phelan et al., 2007). We attributed the lack of impact to two factors: first, the team made recommendations rather than comprehensively managing the patient's care; and second, though co-located, the geriatrician and geriatric nurse practitioner were consultants rather than integral parts of the primary care team. Counsell and colleagues (2007) put a geriatric nurse practitioner and social worker in primary care clinics. Supported by explicit protocols and a multidisciplinary geriatric team, the nurse practitioner and social worker managed complex older patients in concert with the primary care practitioner. This intervention proved to be superior to usual care as measured by quality of care, patient health status, and health care utilization. But the high costs and complexity of the intervention raise important questions about its feasibility and dissemination.

The third intervention, Guided Care, also appears to be effective in improving care and reducing expensive health care utilization, but has the added advantage of being relatively low cost and simple, yet fully integrated with the primary care practice (Boult et al., 2008; Boyd et al., 2007). Because it only involves adding a registered nurse to the practice team, Guided Care may prove to be the most cost-effective way to respond to the needs of multiproblem older patients and their primary care teams. This book is an eminently practical and readable manual to help health care organizations fully consider Guided Care, and, if interested, implement it. It covers every aspect of the intervention from hiring nurses to assuring financial viability.

Until recently, many health care leaders and policy makers questioned whether primary care could ever provide high quality chronic illness or geriatric care. As a consequence, huge sums of money have been diverted to external nurse care management programs on the assumption that they would improve costs and outcomes by working around or bypassing primary care. On the one hand, evidence to date has not confirmed this assumption (Chen et al., 2008; Gravelle et al., 2007). On the other hand, Guided Care (Boult et al., 2008) and the work of Counsell and colleagues (2007) have reassured us that, with additional resources, primary care can provide quality geriatric care. The challenge now is to demonstrate that these interventions can be implemented and effective outside of the externally funded research context, and this book is an important step in that direction.

Edward H. Wagner, MD, MPH, FACP
Director
MacColl Institute for Healthcare Innovation
Group Health Center for Health Studies
1730 Minor Ave., Suite 1290
Seattle, WA 98101–1448
phone 206-287-2877
e-mail wagner.e@ghc.org

REFERENCES

Boult, C., Reider, L., Frey, K., Leff, B., Boyd, C. M., Wolff, J. L., et al. (2008). The early effects of "Guided Care" on the quality of health care for multimorbid older persons: A cluster-randomized controlled trial. *Journals of Gerontology: Medical Sciences, 63(A)(3)*, 321–327.

Boyd, C. M., Boult, C., Shadmi, E., Leff, B., Brager, R., Dunbar, L., et al. (2007). Guided Care for multimorbid older adults. *The Gerontologist, 47(5)*, 697–704.

Chen, A., Brown, R., Esposito, D., Schore, J., & Shapiro, R. (2008). *Report to Congress on the evaluation of Medicare disease management programs* (Mathematica Policy Research, February 14). Retrieved November 24, 2008, from www.mathematica-mpr.com/publications/PDFs/rptcongress_Diseasemgmt.pdf

Counsell, S. R., Callahan, C. M., Clark, D. O., Tu, W., Buttar, A. B., Stump, T. E., et al. (2007). Geriatric care management for low-income seniors: A randomized controlled trial. *Journal of the American Medical Association, 298(22)*, 2623–2633.

Gravelle, H., Dusheiko, M., Sheaff, R., Sargent, P., Boaden, R., Pickard, S., et al. (2007). Impact of case management (Evercare) on frail elderly patients: Controlled before and after analysis of quantitative outcome data. *British Medical Journal (Clinical Research Ed.), 334(7583)*, 31.

Phelan, E. A., Balderson, B., Levine, M., Erro, J. H., Jordan, L., Grothaus, L., et al. (2007). Delivering effective primary care to older adults: A randomized, controlled trial of the senior resource team at Group Health Cooperative. *Journal of the American Geriatrics Society, 55(11)*, 1748–1756.

Preface

This is a book about transformation. Its primary goal is to help medical practices transform their management of patients with several chronic health conditions from the fragmented, depersonalized, inefficient chronic care of today to a new model of coordinated, patient-centered, cost-effective chronic care for tomorrow. We hope that it helps catalyze the transformation of chronic care across America in time to meet the needs of the baby boom generation as its members grow older and experience the challenges of living with chronic diseases.

The book is designed to meet the informational needs of all of the people involved in providing chronic care in outpatient practices: nurses, physicians, practice administrators, office staff members, and executives of health care delivery systems. We encourage everyone to read the entire book, but some may choose to read only those sections that are most relevant to their individual needs. To accommodate these section readers, the book includes certain information in more than one chapter, so that each chapter is comprehensible regardless of whether it is read in sequence or in isolation.

The new model is called "Guided Care." Shaped by the lessons of 30 years of research in chronic care, Guided Care is designed to translate the best available scientific evidence and the most effective health care processes into routine use in most primary care practices (and in some specialty practices) in the United States. Early studies have shown that Guided Care improves the quality of chronic care (Boult et al., 2008; Boyd et al., 2008) and tends to decrease the costs of care, primarily by reducing the use of inpatient facilities (Leff et al., 2008; Sylvia et al., 2008).

Guided Care is not the only model of comprehensive chronic care to show promise recently. Others, which share many features with Guided Care, include Care Management Plus (Dorr, Wilcox, Brunker, Burdon, & Donnelly, 2008), Geriatric Resources and Care for the Elderly (GRACE)

(Counsell et al., 2007), Improving Mood: Promoting Access to Collaborative Treatment (IMPACT) for depression (Unutzer et al., 2002), and team-based care for dementia (Callahan et al., 2006). Each of these models may improve the processes and outcomes of chronic care in the years ahead. Each deserves watching.

This book describes why and how we created the Guided Care model, how it operates, how it affects clinical and financial outcomes, how practice leaders can determine whether Guided Care is right for them and, if it is, how they can adopt and operate it in their practices. Based on the authors' experience in developing and refining Guided Care, the book contains much pragmatic advice and many practical tools, which readers are encouraged to use in their practices. Chapter 7 contains descriptions of and numerous links to other sources of educational and technical assistance for those who wish to adopt the processes of Guided Care in their practices.

Perhaps most valuable, this book describes how practices that participate in the demonstrations of the medical home that are starting in 2009 can obtain supplemental payments to cover the many Guided Care health-related services that are not reimbursed under the contemporary fee-for-service system that pays for most health care in America. The book explains how adopting Guided Care could quickly help transform a struggling practice into a high-functioning medical home that could participate in (and receive supplemental payments from) medical home demonstrations being conducted across the United States by the Centers for Medicare & Medicaid Services (CMS), Blue Cross and Blue Shield plans, other health plans, state Medicaid agencies, and large self-insured employers.

In describing this process, the book points out the similarities and differences between the medical home and the Guided Care models of care. Both models seek to improve the quality and outcomes of care by providing chronically ill patients with easy access to comprehensive, continuous, patient-centered, evidence-based, cost-effective health care. Both rely on health information technology and interdisciplinary teams of physicians, nurses, and other health professionals to deliver care. Both must increase the efficiency of the health care system if they are to become widely adopted and sustainable throughout the decades ahead.

The medical home model, however, is broader than the Guided Care model. As defined by CMS, medical homes must provide certain technological processes—such as the use of electronic registries—that are not required in the Guided Care model. Medical homes also provide supplemental services to all chronically ill Medicare beneficiaries in the practice, whereas Guided Care focuses primarily on the 25% most high-risk beneficiaries. So far, only the Guided Care model has shown improvements in quality of care and trends toward lower health care costs in rigorous scientific studies.

In anticipation of an increasing demand for well-trained Guided Care nurses, the American Nurses Association's American Nurses Credentialing Center (ANA/ANCC) has partnered with the Institute for Johns Hopkins Nursing to create an online course in Guided Care Nursing that will be available at http://www.ijhn.jhmi.edu/contEd_3rdLevel_Class.asp?id=SpecialtyHome&numContEdID=5 in April 2009. Upon completing this course, nurses will be eligible to take an online examination and, if successful, receive a Certificate in Guided Care Nursing from the ANCC. An outline of this course is presented in Appendix A: Online Courses.

The book's Appendix D: Centers for Medicare & Medicaid Services' Medicare Medical Home Demonstration (MMHD) provides many details about CMS's MMHD that specify:

- Which services a practice must provide to be recognized as a fully implemented (Tier 2) medical home.
- The type of health information technology required to be a Tier 2 medical home.
- The diagnoses that make Medicare beneficiaries eligible to participate in the MMHD and, thereby, to generate supplemental payments to participating practices.
- Projections of the amount of supplemental payments a Tier 2 medical home will receive.
- How a practice could use these supplemental payments to cover the costs of providing Guided Care for its sickest patients, providing medical home services for its other chronically ill patients, and acquiring and operating the required health information technology.

We hope you find this book to be clear, concise, pragmatic, helpful, and reasonably up-to-date. Developments related to demonstrations of the medical home, studies of Guided Care, and advancements in chronic care are evolving rapidly, however, so we urge you to visit www.Guided Care.org and the other Web sites provided throughout this book to keep abreast of the latest information.

REFERENCES

Boult, C., Reider, L., Frey, K., Leff, B., Boyd, C. M., Wolff, J. L., et al. (2008). The early effects of "Guided Care" on the quality of health care for multimorbid older persons: A cluster-randomized controlled trial. *Journals of Gerontology: Medical Sciences, 63(A)(3)*, 321–327.

Boyd, C. M., Shadmi, E., Conwell, L. J., Griswold, M., Leff, B., Brager, R., et al. (2008). A pilot test of the effect of Guided Care on the quality of primary care experiences for multimorbid older adults. *Journal of General Internal Medicine, 23(5)*, 536–542.

Callahan, C. M., Boustani, M. A., Unverzagt, F. W., Austrom, M. G., Damush, T. M., Perkins, A. J., et al. (2006). Effectiveness of collaborative care for older adults with Alzheimer's disease in primary care: A randomized controlled trial. *Journal of the American Medical Association, 295(18)*, 2148–2157.

Counsell, S. R., Callahan, C. M., Clark, D. O., Tu, W., Buttar, A. B., Stump, T. E., et al. (2007). Geriatric care management for low-income seniors: A randomized controlled trial. *Journal of the American Medical Association, 298(22)*, 2623–2633.

Dorr, D. A., Wilcox, A. B., Brunker, C. P., Burdon, R. E., & Donnelly, S. M. (2008). The effect of technology supported, multidisease care management on the mortality and hospitalization of seniors. *Journal of the American Geriatric Society, 56(12)*, 2203–2210.

Leff, B., Reider, L., Frick, K., Scharfstein, D., Boyd, C., Frey, K., et al. (2008). "Guided Care" and the cost of complex health care. Manuscript in press.

Sylvia, M. L., Griswold, M., Dunbar, L., Boyd, C., Park, M., & Boult, C. (2008). Guided Care: Cost and utilization outcomes in a pilot study. *Disease Management, 11(1)*, 29–36.

Unutzer, J., Katon, W., Callahan, C. M., Williams, J. W., Jr., Hunkeler, E., Harpole, L., et al. (2002). Collaborative care management of late-life depression in the primary care setting: A randomized controlled trial. *Journal of the American Medical Association, 288(22)*, 2836–2845.

Acknowledgments

This book would not have been possible without the energy, enthusiasm, expertise, conviction, and resources of many, many people.

Our colleagues on the research team who believed in Guided Care from the beginning: Cynthia Boyd, MD, MPH; Rosemarie Brager, PhD, CRNP; Kevin Frick, PhD; Bruce Leff, MD; Jill Marsteller, PhD, MPP; Erin Rand-Giovannotti, Daniel Scharfstein, ScD; Efrat Shadmi, PhD, RN; Martha Sylvia, RN, MSN, MBA; Elizabeth (Ibby) Tanner, PhD, RN; Stephen Wegener, PhD; and Jennifer Wolff, PhD.

The philanthropic organizations, government agencies, and partner organizations that provided support for our randomized controlled trial of Guided Care and encouraged us to disseminate Guided Care into a national model:

The John A. Hartford Foundation, especially Donna Regenstreif, PhD; Amy Berman, RN, BSN; and Christopher Langston, PhD.

The Agency for Healthcare Research and Quality, especially David Meyers, MD; and Claire Kendrick, MSEd, CHES.

The National Institute on Aging, especially Sidney Stahl, PhD.

The Jacob and Valeria Langeloth Foundation, especially Scott Moyer, MPH; and Jennifer Segel, MS.

Kaiser Permanente Mid-Atlantic States, especially Lya Karm, MD; and Carol Groves, RN, MPA.

Johns Hopkins Community Physicians, especially Barbara Cook, MD; and Gary Noronha, MD.

Johns Hopkins HealthCare, especially Patricia Brown, JD; Linda Dunbar, PhD, RN; and Lora Rosenthal, RN, BA, CCM, CMCN.

MedStar Physician Partners, especially Edward Miller, MD.

The Guided Care nurses, who bravely pioneered the original implementation of Guided Care in community-based primary care practices: Cecilia Daub, RN, BSN; Eileen Erbengi, RN, MS; Kathleen Grieve, RN, BSN, MHA, CCM; Carla Jones, RN, BSN, MHS; Rhonda Knotts, RN, BSN, CCM; Melanie Lanier, RN; Julia Mand, RN, BSN; and Michele Phillips, RN, BSN.

The 49 primary care physicians of Johns Hopkins Community Physicians, Kaiser Permanente Mid-Atlantic States, and MedStar Physician Partners who participated in the randomized controlled trial.

The members of the Guided Care Stakeholder Advisory Committee who contributed invaluable advice about making Guided Care diffusible within their national constituencies: Sherry Aliotta, RN, BSN, CCM; Gerard Anderson, PhD; Patricia Archbold, RN, DNSc, FAAN; Sharon Arnold, PhD; Michael Barr, MD, MBA, FACP; Amy Berman RN, BSN; Joseph Berman, MD; John Burton, MD; Jennie Chin Hansen, RN, MS; Charles Chodroff, MD, MBA; Richard Della Penna, MD; Linda Dunbar, PhD, RN; Cynthia Gantt, NC, USN, C-FNP, PhD; Rick Greene, MSW; Kathleen Grieve, RN, BSN, MHA, CCM; Stuart Guterman, MA; David Hellmann, MD, FACP; Christopher Langston, PhD; John Mach, Jr., MD; Joan Marren, RN, MA, MEd; Mathy Mezey, PhD; Michael Montijo, MD, MPH, FACP; Michael O'Dell, MD, MSHA; Donna Regenstreif, PhD; Joan Stanley, RN, PhD, CRNP, FAAN; John Stewart, BS; Robyn Stone, DrPH; Mary Lou Stricklin, RN, MSN, FAAN; and Nancy Whitelaw, PhD.

The busy people who made the time to review drafts of this book and provide thoughtful feedback that proved to enhance the final product significantly: Marilee Aust, BA; Bruce Bagley, MD; Michael Barr, MD, MBA, FACP; John Beilenson, MA; Anna Bergstrom, MSHA; Thomas Bodenheimer, MD, MPH; Barbara Colburn, BA; Teresa Englund, RN, MA; Margaret Gadon, MD, MPH; David Gans, FACMPE; Teresa Garrison, FACMPE; Kathleen Grieve, RN, BSN, MHA, CCM; Carol Groves, RN, MPA; Judi Hertz, PhD, RN; Connie Hofmann, MJ; Rhonda Knotts, RN, CCM; Bruce Leff, MD; Philip Lewer, MSC; Pat Mack, RN, BSN; Terry McGeeney, MD, MBA, FAAFP; Gary Noronha, MD, FACP; Michael O'Dell, MD, MSHA; Michele Phillips, BSN, RN; Lora Rosenthal, RN, BA, CCM, CMCN; David B. Reuben, MD; Julie Sanderson-Austin, RN; Vincenza Snow, MD, FACP; John Swanson, MPH; Edward H. Wagner, MD, MPH, FACP; and Jennifer Wolff, PhD.

To photographers Larry Canner, Donald Battershall, and William Mebane for allowing us to include their beautiful pictures in this book.

And a special thank you to Mari Nicholson, MHS, for her excellent editing and the patience and grace she displayed while pulling this book and its many components together.

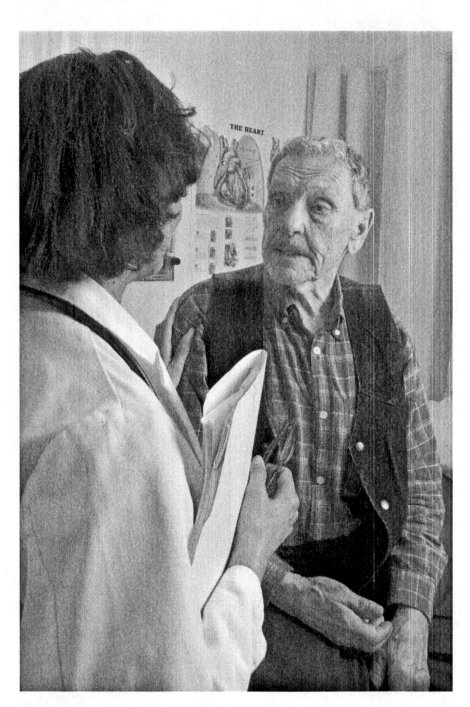

Photo 1.1 Ben Baker, a Guided Care patient.

CREDIT: Photo by Larry Canner.

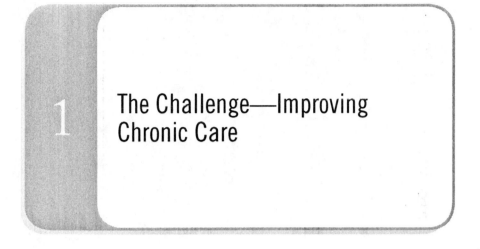

The Challenge—Improving Chronic Care

On January 1, 2011, the American baby boom generation will begin reaching age 65. By 2029, all surviving baby boomers will have entered their golden years, and the population of the United States will include a greater number of older persons than ever before. The U.S. Census Bureau projects that the population of Americans age 65 and older will number 40 million in 2010, nearly 55 million in 2020, and more than 70 million in 2030 (see Figure 1.1).

Some older Americans are healthy, but many others—especially the "oldest old"—have chronic conditions that require complex health care (see Figure 1.2). As the population ages, the number of people with common age-related chronic conditions, such as cancer, hypertension, heart failure, coronary disease, diabetes, stroke, obesity, depression, chronic obstructive pulmonary disease (COPD), and dementia, will rise rapidly. Unless scientists make unprecedented breakthroughs in preventing or curing these conditions soon, the United States will face a pandemic of chronic diseases in the approaching decades.

For 30 years, experts have warned that the United States' health care system, which is focused primarily on caring for acute illnesses and injuries, will be unprepared to provide adequate chronic care for the aging baby boomers (Institute of Medicine, 1978; Institute of Medicine, 1987). Despite these admonitions, America's health care

1

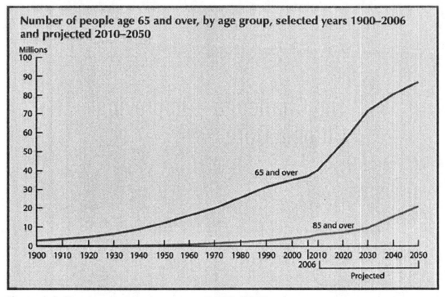

Figure 1.1 Number of older Americans, 1900–2050.

Source: U.S. Census Bureau, Decennial Census, Population Estimates and Projections. Reprinted with permission from the Federal Interagency Forum on Aging-Related Statistics.

policy makers, providers, and insurers have not developed the capacity to provide good chronic care. Its hospitals, nursing homes, outpatient clinics, and home care agencies still operate as uncoordinated "silos" (Institute of Medicine, 2001), much of its physician workforce is inadequately trained in chronic care (Salsberg & Grover, 2006), and the quality and efficiency of chronic care in America remains "far from optimal" (Institute of Medicine, 2001; Salsberg & Grover, 2006; Wenger et al., 2003). In a recent study of health care in six developed nations (the United States, Australia, Canada, Germany, New Zealand, and the United Kingdom), the United States ranked fifth in quality and sixth in access, efficiency, and equity. Nevertheless, per capita health care expenditures were two to three times greater in the United States than in the other nations (see Figure 1.3) (Davis et al., 2007).

The cost of fragmented, chronic care is extraordinarily high. As shown in Figure 1.4, Medicare beneficiaries who have five or more chronic conditions generate two-thirds of all Medicare spending, and

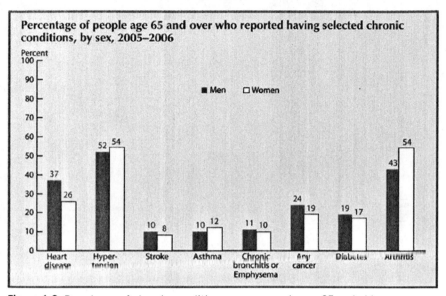

Figure 1.2 Prevalence of chronic conditions among people age 65 and older.

Source: Centers for Disease Control and Prevention, National Center for Health Statistics, National Health Interview Survey. Reprinted with permission from the Federal Interagency Forum on Aging-Related Statistics.

those with four or more chronic conditions account for 80% (Wolff, Starfield, & Anderson, 2002). Much of this spending, which totaled $425 billion in 2007 (Paulson, Chao, Leavitt, Astrue, & Weems, 2008), could be avoided if patients with multiple chronic conditions—such as heart failure, coronary disease, COPD, depression, and diabetes—were monitored regularly, were provided with timely evidence-based ambulatory care, and therefore would require fewer hospital admissions (Wolff et al., 2002). Today, however, Medicare beneficiaries with four or more chronic conditions are 99 times more likely to be admitted to hospitals for "ambulatory care-sensitive conditions" than beneficiaries with only one condition (Wolff et al., 2002). The deteriorating finances of the Part B Medicare program recently mandated congressional intervention, and the trust fund that finances Medicare Part A was projected (before the 2008 recession) to become insolvent by 2019 (Paulson et al., 2008).

Medicare beneficiaries' (and their families') out-of-pocket costs are also high. In 2008, beneficiaries were responsible for paying the costs of:

				Country Rankings	
					1.0–2.66
					2.67–4.33
					4.34–6.0

	AUSTRALIA	CANADA	GERMANY	NEW ZEALAND	UNITED KINGDOM	UNITED STATES
OVERALL RANKING (2007)	3.5	5	2	3.5	1	6
Quality Care	4	6	2.5	2.5	1	5
Right Care	5	6	3	4	2	1
Safe Care	4	5	1	3	2	6
Coordinated Care	3	6	4	2	1	5
Patient-Centered Care	3	6	2	1	4	5
Access	3	5	1	2	4	6
Efficiency	4	5	3	2	1	6
Equity	2	5	4	3	1	6
Long, Healthy, and Productive Lives	1	3	2	4.5	4.5	6
Health Expenditures per Capita, 2004	$2,876*	$3,165	$3,005*	$2,083	$2,546	$6,102

2003 data

Figure 1.3 Health care ratings in six developed nations.

Sources: Reprinted from *Mirror, Mirror on the Wall: An International Update on the Comparative Performance of American Health Care, The Commonwealth Fund,* by K. Davis, C. Schoen, S. C. Schoenbaum, M. M. Doty, A. L. Holmgren, J. L. Kriss, et al., 2007, May. Retrieved July 31, 2008, from http://www.commonwealthfund.org/usr_doc/1027_Davis_mirror_mirror_international_update_final.pdf?section=4039. Calculated by The Commonwealth Fund based on The Commonwealth Fund 2004 International Health Policy Survey, The Commonwealth Fund 2005 International Health Policy Survey of Sicker Adults, The 2006 Commonwealth Fund International Health Policy Survey of Primary Care Physicians, and The Commonwealth Fund Commission on a High Performance Health System National Scorecard.

- Medicare Part A deductibles ($1,024 per benefit period, i.e., the first 60-day period following each admission).
- Medicare Part A co-payments (20% for most services).
- Medicare Part B premiums ($96 to $238 per month, depending on income).
- Medicare Part B deductibles ($135 per year).
- Medicare Part B co-payments (20% for most services).
- Medicare Part D premiums (average of $300 per year).
- Medicare Part D deductibles ($285 per year).
- Medicare Part D co-payments (25% of the first $2,000 after paying the deductible, then 100% of the next $5,000).
- Goods and services not covered by Medicare, such as eyeglasses, hearing aids, dental care, and custodial long-term care at home, in assisted-living facilities, or in nursing homes (15.5% of beneficiaries' income) (Boult, 2006; Neuman, Cubanski, Desmond, & Rice, 2007).

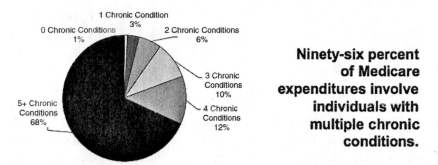

Ninety-six percent of Medicare expenditures involve individuals with multiple chronic conditions.

Figure 1.4 Two-thirds of Medicare spending is for beneficiaries with five or more chronic conditions.

Source: Medicare Standard Analytic File, 2004.

Consider the case history of Mr. Ben Baker, an 81-year-old widowed, retired teacher who has been living on Social Security, a modest pension, and traditional fee-for-service Medicare. Mr. Baker has hypertension, diabetes, heart failure, mild cognitive impairment, osteoarthritis, and depression, for which he takes eight prescription medications each day. His 46-year-old daughter, Helen, who lives across town with her husband and three teenage children, works as an elementary school teacher and is Mr. Baker's primary source of assistance and emotional support. Dr. Lisa Simpson, a primary care physician, sees Mr. Baker approximately every 3 months at routine office visits. Mr. Baker also sees a cardiologist and an orthopedist regularly.

Unfortunately, exacerbations of heart failure have required three episodes of hospital care for Mr. Baker during the past year, each followed by 2 weeks in a skilled nursing facility and several weeks of home health care. Each time he has returned home, Mr. Baker has been weak, depressed, and confused about the medicines he should take and the diet he should follow. Although he has Medicare Parts A, B, and D, his out-of-pocket costs for premiums, deductibles, co-payments, and items not covered by Medicare have totaled more than $5,000 during the past year. Helen, stressed by the many tasks involved in caring for her father and her children, has decreased her teaching (and her income) by 50% and is considering placing her father in a nursing home.

Dr. Simpson is concerned that Mr. Baker may not be safe living alone and that he may not be taking all of his prescribed medications correctly or adhering to his low-salt diet. She is also not sure what medications, diet, or activities Mr. Baker's other doctors have recommended.

Dr. Simpson wishes that she had more time to talk to Mr. Baker and his daughter, but the office visits (for each of which Dr. Simpson receives only $48 from Medicare) last barely long enough for her to do a cursory physical examination and renew the necessary prescriptions.

Older Americans like Mr. Baker need comprehensive, continuous, coordinated primary care, but the availability of primary care in the United States is declining. In 1998, more than half of internal medicine residents chose careers in primary care; now, about 80% become subspecialists or hospitalists (see Figure 1.5) (Bodenheimer, 2006). Similarly, between 1997 and 2008, the number of graduates of U.S. medical schools entering family medicine residencies dropped by 50% (see Figure 1.6). Further exacerbating this trend, many practicing primary care physicians are retiring early as a result of poor remuneration, administrative burdens, and competition from hospitalists, "SNFists" (physicians who practice primarily in skilled nursing facilities), midlevel practitioners, urgent care centers, and "retail clinics" located in large commercial stores.

As this worsening shortage of primary care converges with the growing pandemic of chronic disease, America stands at a dangerous

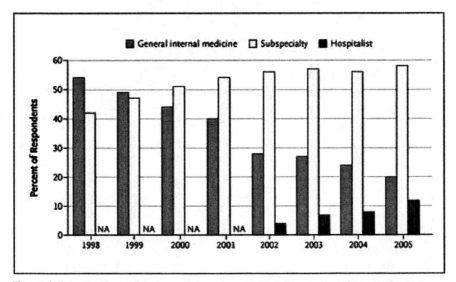

Figure 1.5 Proportions of 3rd-year internal medical residents choosing careers as generalists, subspecialists, and hospitalists.

Source: "Primary Care—Will it Survive?" by T. Bodenheimer, 2006. *The New England Journal of Medicine, 355*(9), 861–864.

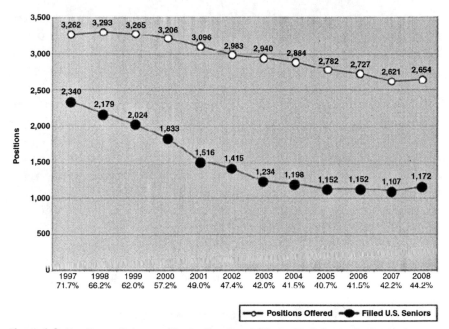

Figure 1.6 Family medicine positions offered and filled with U.S. medical school seniors in March 1997–2008.

Source: Adapted and reprinted with permission from the "National Resident Matching Program," 2008. http://www.aafp.org/online/en/home/residents/match.html. Copyright © 2008 American Academy of Family Physicians. All Rights Reserved.

crossroads (Kane, 2002). If the nation continues on its current course, health care (and health) for people with chronic conditions will deteriorate further and will soon become unsustainably expensive. To change course and confront the looming crisis in chronic care will require courage, leadership, and commitment by national leaders. Within the next 10 years, the United States needs to transform its health care delivery system (Martin et al., 2004) and train its health care professionals to practice the principles of high-quality chronic care (Boult, Christmas, et al., 2008).

So far, attempts to improve the care of Americans with chronic conditions have produced disappointing results. Case management has been used as a complement to primary care to coordinate health care for patients at risk for a variety of undesirable outcomes. Some programs have succeeded in containing costs and increasing patient satisfaction among certain groups of patients, but studies of case management programs that target older patients with multiple chronic conditions have reported little benefit. Significant obstacles to success have included lack of adherence to evidence-based "best practices" and poor coordination with primary care in planning care and sharing information (Pacala et al., 1995).

Disease management programs have sought to improve the quality and outcomes of health care for chronically ill populations defined by specific diagnoses. Disease management programs identify eligible patients from insurance records, compile extensive information about their health, and use it to monitor, educate, empower, and remind (usually by telephone) patients to engage in behaviors that are likely to lead to desirable health outcomes. They also send current clinical information about patients and guidelines for treatment to patients' physicians to encourage them to follow best practices in treating chronic conditions like diabetes and heart failure. Studies of disease management programs for nonelderly patients have reported improvements in outcomes, but most studies of disease management for older patients with several chronic conditions have reported effects on costs that are inconclusive, negative, or difficult to apply to the general population of older persons (Holtz-Eakin, 2004; Ofman et al., 2004).

In the Centers for Medicare & Medicaid Services' large national Medicare Health Support pilot program (Linden & Adler-Milstein, 2008), disease management of beneficiaries with diabetes, heart failure, or COPD failed to achieve the short-term (3-year) cost savings for Medicare that were required for the program to progress from phase one to phase two. Thus, the program stopped providing disease management services in 2008 while debate about the interpretation of its results continued.

Other attempts to improve chronic care have been based on the principle of "pay-for-performance." In these programs, health care providers receive bonus payments if they document (usually on insurance claims) their adherence to preestablished performance standards, such as prescribing appropriate medications and performing appropriate laboratory tests, and if their patients adhere to their recommendations. Studies have confirmed that sufficient payment does induce providers to increase their documented adherence to the agreed upon performance standards (Campbell et al., 2007), but the effects of pay-for-performance on patients' health status, quality of life, and costs of care remain uncertain. Unfortunately, it is very difficult to define, document, and reward excellence in some of the most essential elements of good chronic care, such as care coordination, proactive monitoring, and patient empowerment. As a result, there is serious concern that pay-for-performance incentives for prescribing and testing may lead providers to shift their attention away from care coordination, monitoring, and empowerment. Of equal concern is the possibility that pay-for-performance incentives may discourage physicians from caring for patients who have difficulty adhering to their recommendations.

A conceptual model for improving chronic care is known as the Chronic Care Model (CCM) (see Figure 1.7). This model posits that redesign of the delivery system, enhanced decision support, improved clinical information systems, support for self-management, and better access to and communication with community resources would improve clinical and financial outcomes for people with multiple chronic conditions (Bodenheimer, Wagner, & Grumbach, 2002).

In support of the Chronic Care Model, a review of numerous studies (Bodenheimer, 2003) has shown that improvements in its individual components can improve clinical outcomes and efficiency in outpatient

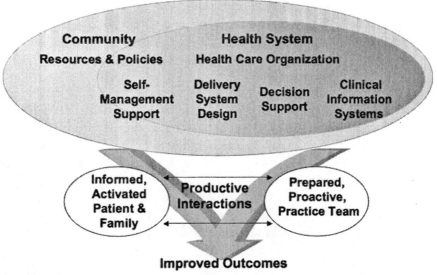

Figure 1.7 Chronic Care Model.

Source: "Chronic Disease Management: What Will It Take to Improve Care for Chronic Illness?" by E. H. Wagner, 1998. *Effective Clinical Practices, 1,* 2–4. The Improving Chronic Illness Care program is supported by The Robert Wood Johnson Foundation with direction and technical assistance provided by Group Health's MacColl Institute for Healthcare Innovation.

settings (Boult et al., 2001; Boult, Green, et al., 2008; Callahan et al., 2006; Cohen et al., 2002; Lorig et al., 2001; Phelan, Williams, Penninx, LoGerfo, & Leveille, 2004; Reuben, Frank, Hirsch, McGuigan, & Maly, 1999; Sommers, Marton, Barbaccia, & Randolph, 2000; Unutzer et al., 2002), in the home (Stuck, Egger, Hammer, Minder, & Beck, 2002), and during transitions between sites of care (Coleman, Parry, Chalmers, & Min, 2006; Naylor et al., 1999). Promising new models of comprehensive chronic care include Care Management Plus (Dorr, Wilcox, Brunker, Burdon, & Donnelly, 2008), and Geriatric Resources and Care for the Elderly (GRACE) (Counsell et al., 2007).

Unfortunately, current insurance reimbursement for such services is very limited, and most general internal medicine (GIM) and family medicine physicians have not been trained to provide them (Darer, Hwang, Pham, Bass, & Anderson, 2004; Rubin, Stieglitz, Vicioso, & Kirk, 2003; Warshaw, Bragg, Brewer, Meganathan, & Ho, 2007). As a result, few medical practices offer these progressive services to their patients.

"Medical home" is a term that denotes health care practices that provide comprehensive, coordinated, continuous care to their patients, including those with chronic conditions that require complex health services. Sometimes referred to as "the advanced medical home" or "the patient-centered medical home," the medical home operationalizes most of the concepts of the Chronic Care Model by incorporating the operative principles of many of the above cited innovations.

In December 2006, the Congress passed and the President signed into law the Tax Relief and Health Care Act (Public Law 109–432), which requires the Centers for Medicare & Medicaid Services (CMS) conduct a 3-year Medicare Medical Home Demonstration (MMHD) in eight states for "high-need Medicare beneficiaries" with "multiple chronic conditions." This law requires CMS to provide care management fees and shared savings (in addition to traditional fee-for-service payments) to qualified medical homes whose physicians and staff members provide at a minimum the following four medical home services:

- Comprehensive, integrated, cross-disciplinary care.
- Evidence-based medicine.
- Tracking patients' health status and providing them with convenient access to care through the use of health information technology.

- Supporting patients' management of their own conditions.

To become recognized as a medical home and, therefore, eligible to participate in the MMHD, practices must provide numerous supplemental services required by CMS (see Appendix D: CMS's Medicare Medical Home Demonstration). Practices have the discretion to decide how they will provide these services; some options include:

- Outsourcing certain services (e.g., contracting with disease management companies that track patients' health status and encourage patients and physicians to adhere to best practice guidelines).
- Training and reorganizing their current physicians and other staff members to provide the supplemental medical home services (e.g., coordinating patients' care and coaching patients and families in self-management).
- Adding to their office staff new clinicians who provide medical home services (e.g., Guided Care nurses [Boyd et al., 2007]).

Outsourcing medical home services is appealing in its simplicity. For example, a practice could contract with a commercial disease management company to monitor its diabetic patients and provide them with health education and reminders to adhere to best practice guidelines in managing their diabetes and other conditions. Disadvantages to this approach include: its disappointing results in the recent Medicare Health Support pilot; its inability to provide "comprehensive, integrated, cross-disciplinary care"; its dissociation from primary care; and its cost to the practice.

Upgrading a practice to the status of medical home by training and redeploying its current physicians and other staff members to provide the required medical home services is another option. An attractive advantage of this approach is economic: the practice would retain all supplemental medical home fees without incurring the costs of hiring additional staff members or paying a third party to provide disease management services.

Disadvantages include the cost, feasibility, and uncertain effectiveness of training and redeploying the practice's physicians and other staff members. Although most physicians could learn to provide medical home services, the costs associated with their learning and providing these services (including the revenue lost by shifting effort from office visits to supplemental medical home services) might exceed the medical home revenue to the practice. The practice's clerical staff and medical assistants would be less expensive to train and redeploy, but the outcomes of assigning such staff to monitor the health status of patients with multiple morbidities, coordinate their care with other providers, and coach them in behavior modification are doubtful and have never been evaluated.

Integrating new clinicians into the office staff is a third option for helping to upgrade practices to medical home status. As described in the next chapter, a specially trained registered nurse, for example, a Guided Care nurse (Boyd et al., 2007), and a licensed practical nurse, could work in partnership with the practice's physicians and other staff members to provide most medical home services to patients with chronic conditions. Advantages to this approach include: simplicity (specialist nurses are responsible for most services), compatibility with current practice (it requires only minor role changes for existing physicians and office staff), efficiency (it aligns nursing roles with nursing skills), accessibility (free online training is available for registered nurses, further explained in Appendix A: Online Courses), improved quality of care (Boult, Reider, et al., 2008; Boyd et al., 2008), high job satisfaction by physicians and nurses (Boult, Reider, et al., 2008), and lower health care costs (Leff et al., 2008; Sylvia et al., 2008). A disadvantage of adding clinicians is the cost of the clinicians, that is, salary, benefits, space, equipment, and travel. Such costs can be covered, however, by the care management fees and shared savings payments made by CMS to qualified medical homes that participate in the MMHD.

The following chapters provide detailed descriptions of how Guided Care operates clinically and financially, how it fits (or not) in different practices, how it affects outcomes, and how traditional practices could provide many medical home services by adopting the Guided Care model.

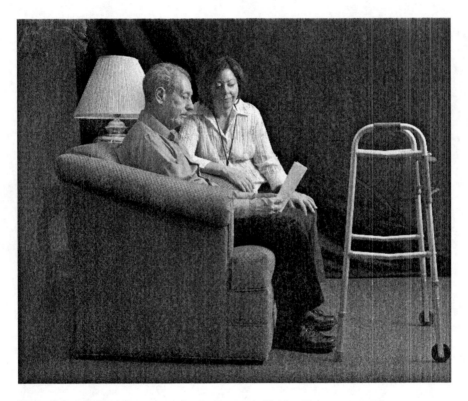

Photo 2.1 A Guided Care nurse conducting an initial health assessment in a patient's home.

Source: Photo courtesy of the John A. Hartford Foundation/Donald Battershall/William Mebane, 2008.

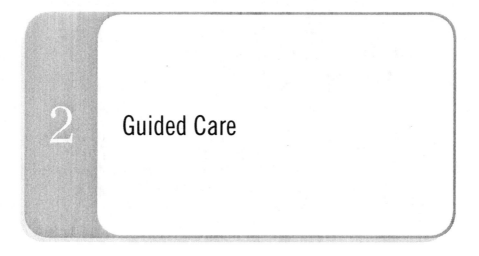

2   Guided Care

To improve chronic care in America, a team of health care professionals convened at Johns Hopkins University in Baltimore to design Guided Care through a series of meetings from 2002 to 2005. The goal was to create a model of care that would provide comprehensive, coordinated, continuing health care to patients who have multiple chronic conditions, a model that could be readily diffused throughout the country (Boyd et al., 2007). The group included physicians, nurses, public health professionals, consumers, educators, behaviorists, policy experts, insurance executives, government officials, and consultants in business and communication. In creating the Guided Care model, the group infused the most current evidence-based guidelines for managing chronic conditions and the most effective principles from case management, disease management, self-management, transitional care, geriatric evaluation, and caregiver support models into primary care.

During 2003–2004, the team conducted a pilot test of Guided Care at a primary care practice in the urban Baltimore community. After creating an electronic health record and constructing a curriculum for preparing nurses to practice Guided Care, they hired and trained a registered nurse to work with two general internists at the pilot practice. The lessons from this 12-month test were instrumental in refining the Guided Care nursing curriculum, the Guided Care model of care, and

Table 2.1

THE EIGHT ACTIVITIES OF THE GUIDED CARE NURSE

ACTIVITY	DESCRIPTION
1	Assessing the patient at home
2	Creating an evidence-based Care Guide
3	Monitoring the patient proactively
4	Empowering the patient; encouraging self-management
5	Coordinating providers of care
6	Smoothing the patient's transitions into and out of the hospital or other facility
7	Educating and supporting caregivers
8	Accessing community resources

the Guided Care electronic health record. The team then conducted a multisite, cluster-randomized trial of Guided Care in the mid-Atlantic United States from 2006–2009.

In the Guided Care model today, a registered nurse collaborates with one or more primary care physicians and their office staff to meet the complex needs of 50 to 60 patients with chronic conditions. The Guided Care nurse, who is based in the primary care office, provides eight essential chronic care services (see Table 2.1), each of which is guided by the patient's priorities and preferences, by scientific evidence, and by an electronic health record. In providing these services, Guided Care practices serve as medical homes for high-need patients with multiple chronic conditions.

EIGHT SERVICES OF GUIDED CARE

Assessing the Patient at Home

Using a standardized questionnaire during a home visit, the Guided Care nurse asks the patient to identify his or her top priorities for optimizing health and quality of life and conducts a 2-hour interview to assess the patient's medical, functional cognitive, affective, psychosocial, nutritional, and environmental status.

The nurse also inquires about the care the patient receives from family caregiver(s), specialist physicians, and community agencies and obtains the patient's signature authorizing the release of medical information. Finally, the nurse gleans supplemental information about the patient's health from the medical records at the primary care office.

Creating an Evidence-Based "Care Guide"

The practice's health information technology merges these individual assessment data with preprogrammed, evidence-based, best-practice management recommendations to create a Preliminary Care Guide that lists medical and behavioral plans for managing and monitoring the patient's chronic conditions. A sample, Resource 2A· Preliminary Care Guide, is located at the end of this chapter.

In a subsequent 20-minute meeting, the Guided Care nurse and the primary care physician discuss and modify this guide to align it with the unique circumstances of the individual patient. During their conversation, the nurse makes handwritten comments on the Preliminary Care Guide to reflect their joint decisions.

The Guided Care nurse then discusses the modified Preliminary Care Guide with the patient and caregiver and modifies it further for consistency with their preferences, priorities, and intentions. The nurse then enters these revisions into the practice's health information technology.

The final Care Guide, which is then produced by the health information technology, provides all involved health care professionals with a concise summary of the patient's health status and health-related plans. A sample of this form, Resource 2B: Care Guide, is found at the end of this chapter.

The nurse then creates and prints a patient-friendly version of the Care Guide for the patient and caregiver. This Action Plan (see Resource 2C: Action Plan), which is written in large type and lay language, is displayed prominently in the home to remind the patient to take medications, observe dietary restrictions, participate in appropriate physical activity, monitor physiological parameters such as weight and blood pressure, and follow up with health professionals on schedule. The Action Plan also denotes symptoms and situations (i.e., red flags) that should prompt the patient or caregiver to call the nurse's cellular phone or go to the local hospital's emergency department.

Monitoring the Patient Proactively

With daily reminders generated by the health information technology, the Guided Care nurse monitors each patient proactively at least monthly, usually by telephone, to evaluate adherence to the Action Plan and to detect and address emerging problems promptly. In addition, the patient and caregiver are encouraged to call the Guided Care nurse's cellular phone if they have questions or concerns. When health-related problems emerge, the Guided Care nurse discusses them with the patient's primary care physician and implements appropriate actions. On nights and weekends when the nurse is off duty, patients' and caregivers' calls are directed to the primary care practice's usual answering/on-call system.

Empowering the Patient; Encouraging Self-Management

As described in Appendix A: Online Courses, Guided Care nurses are taught to use the principles and techniques of motivational interviewing for healthy behavior (Bennett et al., 2005; Rollnick, Mason, & Butler, 1999), which are based on the transtheoretical model of change (Prochaska & DiClemente, 1984). Guided Care nurses use motivational interviewing to identify obstacles and develop strategies that empower patients to adopt healthy behaviors and to participate actively in their health care according to their specific Action Plans. Recognizing that patients move through various stages of making health-behavior changes, Guided Care nurses identify patients' health-related goals and preferences, express empathy, clarify discrepancies between current behavior and health goals, avoid arguing, provide health education, and support patients' self-efficacy.

To improve patients' self-efficacy in managing their chronic conditions, the Guided Care nurse refers most patients to a local chronic disease self-management (CDSM) course. The curriculum of this course was developed at Stanford University and is now available for free or at a nominal cost in many communities (Lorig & Holman, 2003). Its six, 2-hour 30-minute sessions are facilitated by trained lay leaders (see http://www.healthyaging programs.org/content.asp?sectionid=32&elementid=483). In these group sessions, patients learn to create and use Action Plans, which they use with the Guided Care nurse to reach their health-related goals. Information needed to refer patients to these local courses is available from each regional Area Agency on Aging (see www.eldercare.gov/Eldercare/Public/

Home.asp). The National Council on the Aging (www.ncoa.org) plans to offer an online version of this course in 2009.

Coordinating Providers of Care

In concert with the other members of the practice team, the Guided Care nurse coordinates the efforts of the many health care professionals who treat Guided Care patients—in primary care, emergency departments, hospitals, rehabilitation facilities, specialists' offices, nursing homes, and in the home. The Guided Care nurse's primary tool for coordinating care is the Care Guide. The nurse provides this concise up-to-date summary of each Guided Care patient's history, conditions, current therapy and plans, recent parameters, and advance directives to all other involved health care providers. Although the nurse cannot require other providers to follow the Care Guide, most professionals regard it as a convenient basis for further action.

The Guided Care nurse monitors the actions of the other providers (e.g., prescriptions, tests, referrals, and recommendations) through the patients, the caregivers, consultation reports, and calls to the other providers (facilitated by faxing the patient's signed authorization for release of information). Based on this monitoring, the nurse updates the Care Guide and the Action Plan as often as necessary to reflect changes in the patient's health status and plans.

Smoothing the Patient's Transitions Into and Out of Hospitals and Other Facilities

Patients are strongly encouraged to contact their Guided Care nurses before or during all admissions to emergency departments and hospitals. As discussed in chapter 5, notices from the practice's physicians and office staff, as well as local hospitals, also help inform the nurse promptly when patients are admitted. Upon learning of a patient's admission, the Guided Care nurse:

- Provides health care professionals in the inpatient setting with complete, current clinical information and explains the Guided Care nurse's role in assisting the patient after the patient has been discharged. Usually, the nurse hand delivers the patient's Care Guide during an on-site conversation with a hospital nurse within the first 24 hours of admission.

- Visits the patient and communicates with the hospital staff (e.g., nurses, physicians, social workers, case managers, and discharge coordinators) throughout the hospital stay. This provides opportunities to optimize the patient's post-hospital care by informing the hospital staff of the patient's unique home circumstances and by monitoring inpatient changes in the patient's medications and other treatments (facilitated by presenting the patient's signed authorization for release of information).
- Prepares the patient and family for the transition out of the hospital.
- Visits the patient at home 1 to 2 days after discharge to evaluate the patient's recovery, to adjudicate medications, and to ensure that the patient and caregiver know what they should be doing, which circumstances should cause concern, and whom to call for advice.
- Briefs the primary care physician about the patient's hospital course and current status, and ensures that the patient sees the primary care physician soon after discharge.

Educating and Supporting Caregivers

For the family or other unpaid caregivers of patients with functional impairment or difficulty performing health-related tasks, the Guided Care nurse offers three forms of assistance: initial assessment of the caregiver, information and advice about caregiving, and ad hoc telephone consultation. The information and advice about caregiving, which is covered in the Guided Care Nursing course (see Appendix A: Online Courses), includes practical guidance for providing care to loved ones, as well as lists of community-based resources, including support groups that are available to caregivers.

Accessing Community Resources

In concert with the practice's office staff, the Guided Care nurse maintains a database of the resources in the local community that may be helpful to people with chronic conditions. Based on the initial assessment of the patient's and caregiver's needs, the nurse informs the patient and caregiver of the availability of these resources and suggests that they consider using them (or, when necessary, makes calls to appropriate agencies on their behalf). The Guided Care nurse may suggest, for

Table 2.2

GUIDED CARE NURSE'S TYPICAL TIME ALLOCATION IN A 40-HOUR WEEK	
GUIDED CARE ACTIVITY	**HOURS PER WEEK (AVERAGE)**
Assessing new patients and caregivers (to replenish caseload after patients die or move away)	3.5
Scheduled monitoring and coaching	8.0
Coordinating transitions between sites and providers of care	4.0
Documenting activities and updating Care Guides and Action Plans	8.0
Addressing emerging issues with patients and caregivers	4.0
Communicating with primary care physicians (PCP) and other providers	3.0
Accessing community resources	0.5
Facilitating caregiver support groups	1.0
Other administrative tasks, including attending meetings, traveling to and from patients' homes and hospitals, responding to e-mail, interacting with practice staff, and organizing patient charts	8.0
Total hours per week	**40.0**

example, that the patient or caregiver contact a transportation service, the Meals on Wheels Association of America, the local Area Agency on Aging, or the local Alzheimer's Association.

The average amount of time spent by Guided Care nurses on specific activities during a typical 40-hour, 5-day week are shown in Table 2.2.

DIFFERENCES BETWEEN GUIDED CARE AND OTHER RELATED CARE MODELS

Guided Care was derived from several previously tested models of care for people with chronic conditions, including case management, disease management, self-management, geriatric evaluation and management, transitional care, and caregiver support. Thus, it shares features with each of these models, but its aggregate scope of clinical activities is broader than the scope of any one of them. Other important differences are:

- The location of Guided Care nurses in the primary care office, which facilitates communication and teamwork involving the nurse, physicians, and office staff.
- The systematic targeting of patients who have multiple chronic conditions.
- The depth and intensity of the relationships among the nurse, the patient, the caregiver, the office staff, and the primary care physician.
- The longitudinal nature of Guided Care, that is, most patients receive it for life.
- Guided Care nurses' rigorous training (through the Guided Care Nursing course), knowledge (as demonstrated on the Guided Care Nursing examination), and focus on selected clinical activities that have been shown to improve outcomes of care.
- The use of health information technology to provide evidence-based care plans, reminders, and decision support.

THE TOOLS OF GUIDED CARE

Health Information Technology

In studies at Johns Hopkins University, Guided Care nurses have used an in-house electronic health record. Most of the functions of this electronic record are now available within health information technologies that are available for purchase or licensing. Specific information about the functions and the costs of many of these electronic health records is available at www.transformed.com/MedicalHomeMarketplace, www.acponline.org, and www.centerforhit.org.

After the nurse enters data from each patient's initial assessment, the practice's technology integrates current evidence-based recommendations for managing the patient's chronic conditions into a personalized Care Guide, which supplements the patient's other medical records. The nurse also uses this technology to check for potential adverse interactions in the patient's drug regimen, to update the Care Guide, to monitor and coach the patient, to provide reminders of needed care, and to document all contacts with patients, caregivers, and health care providers.

Predictive Model

Identifying the patients who are most likely to benefit from Guided Care (i.e., those with multimorbidity, complex health care needs, and high health care expenditures) is crucial to the cost-effectiveness of Guided Care. Insurers and provider organizations can use the public domain hierarchical condition category (HCC) predictive model (www.cms.hhs. gov/MedicareAdvtgSpecRateStats/06_Risk_adjustment.asp) to analyze the insurance claims for care of all older patients in the practice's panel during the previous year. The HCC predictive model uses administrative data and diagnoses from insurance claims to compute a patient's probability of using health care heavily in the future. The 20% to 25% of older patients in the panel who have the highest estimated need for complex health care in the future are selected for Guided Care. No high-risk patients are excluded because of a condition (e.g., dementia) or place of residence (e.g., nursing home), although some cognitively impaired patients are unable to participate fully in chronic disease self-management. Although clinicians are also capable of identifying patients with multimorbidity, electronic predictive models can identify such patients more objectively, consistently, and efficiently (Institute for Health Policy Solutions, 2005).

THE EFFECTS OF GUIDED CARE

Guided Care is popular with patients, caregivers, physicians, and nurses (see Table 2.3). A pilot study and a multisite cluster-randomized controlled trial (see Table 2.4) showed that it also improves the quality of chronic care as rated by patients on validated survey instruments (Boult, Reider, et al., 2008; Boyd et al., 2008). During a pilot test (Sylvia et al., 2008) and the first 8 months of a multisite, cluster-randomized trial (Leff et al., 2008), patients who received Guided Care tended to generate lower expenditures for health insurers, mostly by using less inpatient care. The longer-term effects of Guided Care on these and other important outcomes will be reported after the randomized trial is completed in June 2009.

Table 2.3

CHANGES IN PHYSICIAN SATISFACTION WITH THEIR CHRONIC CARE BETWEEN BASELINE AND 1 YEAR LATER

	PHYSICIANS WHO PROVIDED GUIDED CARE ($N = 18$)	PHYSICIANS WHO PROVIDED USUAL CARE ($N = 20$)	P VALUE[a]
Communicating with patients	0.11	−0.42	0.047
Communicating with caregivers	0.39	−0.11	0.066
Educating caregivers	0.50	−0.34	0.008
Motivating patients	0.39	−0.40	0.006
Knowing all patients' medications	0.29	−0.18	0.034

[a]t test.
Note. Positive scores indicate higher satisfaction after 1 year than at baseline. Negative scores indicate lower satisfaction after 1 year than at baseline (Boult, Reider, et al., 2008).

Physicians have expressed appreciation and enthusiasm for Guided Care, saying that Guided Care improves the quality of the patients' chronic care, especially the communication and coordination among providers. One physician said, "The Guided Care Nurse was able to inform me about the details of my patient's hospitalization because she had a conversation with the hospital physician and his staff about how they made the diagnosis and how it affected the treatment plan. [Also], post-discharge, she helped me to get the records necessary for me to decide how long the patient needed antibiotics and what the appropriate follow up should be."

Similarly, Guided Care nurses enjoy their work, stating, "This is the way nursing should be practiced: a partnership with physicians, really knowing and helping your patients and families. It's the type of work that attracted me to nursing in the first place." Not surprisingly, most patients and families are very happy with Guided Care: "It's like having a nurse in the family."

Table 2.4

THE QUALITY OF HEALTH CARE IN GUIDED CARE (GC) AND USUAL CARE (UC) GROUPS AFTER 6 MONTHS

PATIENT ASSESSMENT OF CHRONIC ILLNESS CARE (PACIC) SCALES	ADJUSTED ODDS RATIO	95% CONFIDENCE INTERVAL	P VALUE
Goal setting	2.37	1.53–3.67	<0.001
Coordination of care	2.25	1.27–3.97	0.005
Decision support	1.51	1.08–2.10	0.014
Problem solving	1.35	0.95–1.93	0.096
Patient activation	1.06	0.74–1.52	0.763
Aggregate quality	2.03	1.22–3.39	0.006

Note. Adjusted for participants' baseline sociodemographic characteristics (i.e., age, race, sex, educational level, economic status, habitation status, health status [i.e., HCC score], functional ability [i.e., SF-36 PCS and MCS scores], baseline patient assessment of chronic illness care [PACIC] score, satisfaction with health care, and practice site) (Boult, Reider, et al., 2008).

Family caregivers report significantly less strain if their loved ones receive Guided Care (Wolff et al., in press). Other outcomes, such as patients' quality of life and functional independence, and practices' operational flow and dynamics are currently under study.

REQUIREMENTS FOR ADOPTING GUIDED CARE

Discussed in detail in the following chapter, a practice that wishes to become a Guided Care medical home must meet certain criteria.

- Panel size: Large enough to contain 50 to 60 patients with several chronic conditions. Panels of at least 300 Medicare patients are usually sufficient.
- Office space: A small, private, centrally located office for the nurse.
- Health information technology: A locally installed electronic health record or a Web-based health information technology system can provide the necessary support.

■ Commitment: By the practice's physician(s) and office staff members to work collaboratively with the Guided Care nurse.

PRACTICAL CONSIDERATIONS

Guided Care produces crucial improvements in chronic care. It also generates significant costs for the practice: the nurse's salary and benefits, office space, equipment, communication services, and travel costs. To adopt Guided Care, a practice must be confident that it will receive a revenue stream that will offset these costs. Chapter 7 estimates the costs of Guided Care and describes sources of offsetting revenue and the business case for adopting Guided Care.

Although this book provides an introduction to Guided Care, many practices will desire more assistance in getting started. Chapter 7 provides details about courses and technical assistance that are available online, by telephone, and in person. Appendix A: Online Courses provides information for registered nurses who may wish to become Guided Care nurses and for physicians who wish to practice effectively in medical homes.

RESOURCE 2A: PRELIMINARY CARE GUIDE

Health Problems of Greatest Importance to Patient

Constant aching back
Tired all the time
Can't move my bowels

GCN Impressions

Chaotic medicine cabinet; environment unsafe because of disability

PCP Impressions

Patient will say she wants to make changes, but has difficulty following through. Has solid caregiver support.

Chronic Conditions

Condition	Descriptive information
Constipation	2 BMs perweek, Abdominal Bloating 7 times per week
Depression	Onset - 1998, 0 drinks per week, GDS - 10/15, Suicidal Activity
Disability	Difficulty bathing, difficulty doing housework, difficulty shopping, difficulty traveling
Osteoarthritis	Pain Score - 71/10, uses walker (not functional), area(s) most affected - Hip, Knee, Spine
Other	Condition Notes - cataracts
Other	Condition Notes - spinal stenosis
Persistent Pain	Pain Score - 71/10, uses walker (not functional), cause - arthritis, most affected - Hip, Knee, Back

Important allergies and other adverse reactions to medications

Substance	Reaction	Year
Penicillin	Difficulty breathing	1972

Chronic medicine

Name	Dose	Rte	Freq	Discrepancy	Nature	Reason	Potential Interaction	Change
Nabumetone	750 mg	PO	BID	N			none	—
Oxycodone and Acetaminophen	5/325 mg	PO	BID	Y	Not taking at all	Side effect(s)	none	D/C
Tramadol	NA	PO	PRN	Y	Not prescribed for patient	Borrowed from another person	Sertraline	D/C
Bisacodyl	NA	PO	PRN	Y	Not prescribed for patient	Other	Sertraline	D/C
Sertraline	50 mg	PO	QHS	N			Tramadol, Bisacodyl	—
Acetaminophen	325 mg	PO	BID	N			none	650 mg po QID
Psyllium	1 tsp	PO	QD	Y	Not prescribed for patient	Other	none	approve

Overall Adherence: Poor

(Continued)

RESOURCE 2A: PRELIMINARY CARE GUIDE *(Continued)*

Management

Diet: Recommended by Guideline		Actual Diet
☐ Constipation	High-fiber diet: bran, fruits, vegetables	None
☐ Constipation	32+ oz of oral fluid intake daily	
☐ Osteoarthritis	Gradual weight-reducing (if obese)	
☐ Other:		

Physical Activity: Recommended by Guideline		Actual Physical Activity
☐ Copnstipation	Regular mild-moderate exercise	None
☐ Depression	Regular mild-moderate exercies	
☐ Osteoarthritis	Regular mild-moderate exerciese for flexibility, strength, and/or endurance	
☐ Persistent Pain	Regular mild-moderate exercies	
☐ Other:		

Other: Recommednded by Guideline		Actual Other
☐ Depression	Remove exposure to contributing factors: medications, alcohol	None
☐ Persisten Pain	Treat underlying cause of pain, if possible	
☐ Other:		

Monitoring: Recommednded by Guideline

☐ Depression	Patient or caregiver to report increased symptoms of depression
☐ Depression	Regular visits with mental health professional
☐ Persistent Pain	Maintain a record of pain level daily
	Proactive Followup: __pt__ to call __GCN__ every _1_ month(s)
	Primary Care office visits every _3_ month(s)
☐ Other:	

Specialist: Recommended by Guideline		Actual Specialist
☐ Other:		None

Referral: Recommended by Guideline

☐ Depression	Counseling by mental health professional
☐ Osteoarthritis	Education and counseling
☐ Other:	

RESOURCE 2A: PRELIMINARY CARE GUIDE *(Continued)*

Health maintenance options (some may not be appropriate for this patient)

Immunizations: ☐ flu shot 11/1   ☐ pneumococcal vaccination [11/09] (5 yrs from prev, 2004)

Screening: ☐ stool blood [11/09] (1 yr from   ☐ lipid profile [11/09] (1 yr from prev, 12/2008) prev, 12/2008)

☐ colon/sigmoid-oscopy [11/09] (5 yrs from prev, 12/2004)

Women:

☐ mammogram [11/09] (2 yrs from prev, 12/2007)   ☐ TSH [11/09] (1 yr from prev, 12/2008)

☐ hip/spine DXA [11/09] (2 yrs from prev, 2/2007)

☐ Annual check-up with physician for immunizations, screening, self-care (diet, exercise)

☐ Complete DPOAHC or health care agent   ☐ Put DPOAHC or agent document on chart

☐ Rec. home modification: lighting, hazards for falling, telephone access, smoke detector(s)

☐ Coaching for risk reduction and self-management   ☐ Smoking cessation program (currently smoking)

☐ Chronic Disease Self-Management (CDSM) course   ☐ PT referral

☐ Hearing eval by audiologist (hearing screen score   Fail)   ☐ OT referral

☐ Nutrition eval by dietician (nutrition screen score = 3+/21)   ☐ Other: _____

(Continued)

RESOURCE 2A: PRELIMINARY CARE GUIDE *(Continued)*

Background Information

Recent providers

Name	Discipline	Phone Type	Phone Nbr	Email
Maureen Benchaim	Family Practice	Business	(202) 891-4233	mbenchaim@med.com
Willard Choi	Ophthalmology	Business	(202) 323-0071	wchoi@med.com
Richard Payne	Orthopedic Surgery	Business	(202) 991-1123	rpayne@med.com

Services being used

Service	Agency	Phone Type	Phone Nbr	Notes
Service (Rides)	Metro Mobility	Business	(202) 954-1300	

Devices

Walker (Not functional)

Hospitalizations in the past 2 years

Date	Details
7/14/2008	Hospitalization. 3 day adm. to County General Hospital to evaluate/treat increased back pain

Spirituality (in relation to health)

Religion	Catholic
Religion's importance in health	High

Indicators

Indicator	Value
Alcohol Use (Drinks/Week)	0
CAGE Assessment Score	0
Tobacco Use (Packs/Day)	0

DPOAHC or health care agent

Name	Relationship	Phone Type	Phone Nbr
Marsha Palmer	Care Giver (Primary)	Home	(202) 326-1126

Contacts

Name	Relationship	Phone Type	Phone Nbr
Linda Palmer	Daughter	Home	(202) 291-7059
Robert Palmer	Son	Home	(202) 338-1971
John Palmer	Son	Home	(202) 234-2630
Eileen Novak	Guided Care Nurse	Business	(202) 816-6798

Caregiver Information

Name: Marsha Palmer; Age: 55; Co-resident: No; Driving status: I drive; Stress level: Low; Employment: Full Time

RESOURCE 2A: PRELIMINARY CARE GUIDE *(Continued)*

Insurance coverage

Carrier	Policy Nbr	Effective Date	Notes
Medicare A	217034521A	07/17/2006	
Medicare B	217034521A	07/17/2006	
Medicaid	033456987	07/17/2006	
Medicare D	265984589A	07/17/2008	

Financial strain related to using health services

Financial strain for hospital/home care?	Yes
Financial strain for physician services/tests?	No
Financial strain for prescription medications?	No

RESOURCE 2A: CARE GUIDE TARGETS AND RED FLAGS

Condition	Targets	Red Flags
General	Adherence to medications	Almost out of any medication
Constipation	Three soft stools per week Minimal straining Minimal bloating	Abdominal pain Nausea and vomiting Rectal bleeding
Depression	Depression does not limit ability to do desired activities.	↑ symptoms ↑ use of alcohol Suicidal thoughts
Osteoarthritis	OA pain does not limit ability to do desired activities.	↑ pain
Persistent pain	Pain does not limit ability to do desired activities.	↑ pain New/increased confusion Falls

RESOURCE 2A: CARE GUIDE TARGETS AND
RED FLAGS *(Continued)*

Constipation

Guidelines

<u>Diet</u>

32+ oz of oral fluid intake daily
High-fiber diet: bran, fruits, vegetables

<u>Education</u>

Discuss the range of "normal" bowel function

<u>Medications</u>

Judicious, step-care use of laxatives: fiber/bulk, stimulant, osmotic, enema
Minimize use of constipating medications: opiates, iron, diuretics, antacids, Ca-blockers,
anti-cholinergics, anti-histamines, anti-psychotics, cholestyramine, clonidine

<u>Physical Activity</u>

Regular mild-moderate exercise

Targets

Minimal bloating
Minimal Straining
Soft stools per week = 3

Red Flags

Abdominal pain
Nausea and vomiting
Rectal bleeding

Background Information

Year of onset	2003
Straining occurrences per week	7
Incomplete evacuations per week	2
Abdominal bloating occurrences per week	7
# of BMs per week	2
Typical consistency	Hard

Current Management

Daily oral hydration	32+ oz

Most Recent Results

<u>Measure</u>	<u>Date</u>	<u>Results</u>

(Continued)

RESOURCE 2A: CARE GUIDE TARGETS AND
RED FLAGS (Continued)

Depression

Guidelines

Medications
SSRI: sertaline (Zoloft), paroxetine (Paxil), citalopram (Celexa), escitalopram (Lexapro)

Monitoring
Patient or caregiver to report increased symptoms of depression
Regular visits with mental health professional

Other
Remove exposure to contributing factors: medications, alcohol

Physical Activity
Regular mild-moderate exercise

Referral
Counseling by mental health professional

Targets

Depression limits the ability to do desired activities = No

Red Flags

Increased symptoms of depression
Increased use of alcohol
Suicidal ideation

Background Information

Year of onset	1998
History of depression	Yes
Suicidal activity	No
Recent losses or crises	No

Previous Management

Medicine	depression meds
Medicine - reason for stopping or not starting	sick to stomach

Most Recent Results

Measure	Date	Results
Alcohol use (drinks/week)	7/2008	0

RESOURCE 2A: CARE GUIDE TARGETS AND RED FLAGS *(Continued)*

Disability

Guidelines

Targets

Red Flags

Background Information

Year of onset	2000
Physical barrier to home entry	stairs to 2nd floor apt
Physical barrier inside home	none
Resource used to manage transportation/walking outside home	Person
Resource used to manage shopping	Person
Resource used to manage light housework	Person
Resource used to manage bathing	Person
Unsafe stove	no

Most Recent Results

Measure	Date	Results

(Continued)

RESOURCE 2A: CARE GUIDE TARGETS AND
RED FLAGS *(Continued)*

Osteoarthritis

Guidelines

Diet

Gradual weight-reducing (if obese)

Medications

For chronic pain: acetaminophen 650-1000 mg po TID-QID
For exacerbations of pain: Add NSAID and/or capsaicin cream temporarily. Avoid NSAID in PUD,
CHF, HTN, and renal insufficiency.
If acetaminophen, NSAID, and capsaicin not effective, add an opiod temporarily. Observe for
adverse effects of opioids: cogn constipation.

Physical Activity

Regular mild-moderate exercise for flexibility, strength, and/or endurance

Referral

Education and counseling

Targets

Pain limits person's ability to do desired activities = No

Red Flags

Persistently increased pain

Background Information

Year of onset	1991
Area(s) most affected	Hip, Knee, Spine
Functional limitation by arthritis	A lot

Previous Management

Medicine	Vioxx
Medicine - reason for stopping or not starting	dangerous

Most Recent Results

Measure	Date	Results
BUN	2/2006	30
Creatinine	2/2006	1.5
X-ray - Joint/Bone	2/2007	normal

RESOURCE 2A: CARE GUIDE TARGETS AND RED FLAGS (Continued)

Persistent Pain

Guidelines

Education

Encourage pain education, self-management, and cognitive-behavioral therapy

Medications

Acetaminophen (e.g., Tylenol) 650-1000 mg po TID-QID. Do not exceed 4g per 24 hrs. Reduce dose 50-75% in liver disease or alcoholism.

Avoid: propoxyphere (Darvon), tramadol (Ultram), methadone (Dolophine)

For exacerbations of pain: Add NSAID and/or capsaicin cream temporarily. Avoid NSAID in PUD, CHF, HTN, and renal insufficiency.

If Acetaminophen is not effective, add a non-acetylated salicylate: salsalate (e.g., Disalcid), trisalicylate (e.g., Trilisate)

If an opioid is not effective, add an adjuvant: nortriptyline (e.g., Aventil) if patient is depressed, or carbamazepine (Tegretol) i neuropathic.

If non-acetylated salicylate is not effective, add an opioid: oxycodone (OxyContin), morphine (MSContin), transdermal fentan (Duragesic).

If taking an opioid, protect against and monitor for serious adverse side effects: constipation, impairment in cognition (car crs gait, balance (falls).

Monitoring

Maintain a record of pain level daily

Other

Treat underlying cause of pain, if possible

Physical Activity

Regular mild-moderate exercise

Targets

Pain limits person's ability to do desired activities = No

Red Flags

Confusion

Constipation

Falls

Persistently increased pain

Background Information

Year of onset	1998
Description	Aching
Most affected	Hip, Knee, Back
Cause	Arthritis
Pain limits	Daily activities, Social activities, Quality of life

(Continued)

RESOURCE 2A: CARE GUIDE TARGETS AND
RED FLAGS *(Continued)*

Current Management

Physical treatments   Heat, Salve _____

Previous Management

Medicine   pain meds _____

Medicine - Reason for stopping or not   causes constipation
starting   _____

Most Recent Results

Measure	Date	Results
ALT	2/2006	44
AST	2/2006	50

RESOURCE 2B: CARE GUIDE

Chronic Conditions

Condition	Descriptive information
Constipation	2 BMs per week, abdominal bloating 7 times per week
Depression	Onset - 1998, 0 drinks per week, GDS - 10/15, suicidal activity
Disability	Difficulty bathing, difficulty doing housework, difficulty shopping, difficulty traveling
Osteoarthritis	Pain score - 7/10, uses walker (not functional), Area(s) most affected - Hip, Knee, Spine
Other	Condition notes - cataracts
Other	Condition notes - spinal stenosis
Persistent Pain	Pain score - 7/10, uses walker (not functional), Cause - arthritis, most affected - Hip, Knee, Back

Chronic Prescription Medications

Name	Dose	Rte	Freq
Nabumetone	750 mg	PO	BID
Oxycodone and Acetaminophen	5/325 mg	PO	BID
Tramadol	NA	PO	PRN
Bisacodyl	NA	PO	PRN
Sertraline	50 mg	PO	QHS
Acetaminophen	325 mg	PO	BID
Psyllium	1 tsp	PO	QD

Overall Adherence: Poor

Important allergies and adverse reactions to medications

Substance	Reaction	Year
Penicillin	Difficulty breathing	1972

Management

Diet

32+ oz of oral fluid intake daily

High-fiber diet: bran, fruits, vegetables

Monitoring

Maintain a record of pain level daily

PCP office visits every 3 months

Pt to call GCN every month

Regular visits with mental health professional

Physical Activity

Regular mild-moderate exercise for flexibility, strength, and/or endurance

(Continued)

RESOURCE 2B: CARE GUIDE *(Continued)*

Health Maintenance Due

Immunizations: pneumococcal vaccination [11/2009]
Tests: colon/sigmoid-oscopy [11/2009]   hip/spine DXA [11/2009]   lipid profile [11/2009]
     mammogram [11/2009]

Contacts

Name	Relationship	Phone Type	Phone Nbr
Linda Palmer	Daughter	Home	(202) 291-7059
Robert Palmer	Son	Home	(202) 338-1971
John Palmer	Son	Home	(202) 234-2630
Eileen Novak	Guided Care Nurse	Business	(202) 816-6798

Caregiver Information

Name: Marsha Palmer; Age: 55; Co-resident: No; Driving status: I drive; Stress level: Low; Employment: Full Time

DPOAHC or Health Care Agent

Full Name	Relationship	Phone Type	Phone Nbr
Marsha Palmer	Care Giver (Primary)	Home	(202) 326-1126

Hospitalizations in the Past 2 Years

Date	Details
7/14/2008	Hospitalization. 3 day adm. to County General Hospital to evaluate/treat increased back pain

RESOURCE 2B: CARE GUIDE *(Continued)*

Supporting Information

Recent Providers

Name	Discipline	Phone Type	Phone Nbr	Email
Maureen Benchaim	Family Practice	Business	(202) 891-4233	mbenchaim@med.com
Willard Choi	Ophthalmology	Business	(202) 323-0071	wchoi@med.com
Richard Payne	Orthopedic Surgery	Business	(202) 991-1123	rpayne@med.com

Services Being Used

Service	Agency	Phone Type	Phone Nbr	Notes
Service (Rides)	Metro Mobility	Business	(202) 954-1300	

Referrals Planned

Education and counseling

Devices Being Used

Spirituality (in relation to health)

Religion	Catholic
Religion's importance in health	High

Insurance Coverage

Carrier	Policy Nbr	Effective Date	Notes
Medicare A	217034521A	07/17/2006	
Medicare B	217034521A	07/17/2006	
Medicaid	033456987	07/17/2006	
Medicare D	265984589A	07/17/2008	

Financial Strain Related to Using Health Services

Financial Strain for Hospital/Home Care?	Yes
Financial Strain for Physician Services/Tests?	No
Financial Strain for Prescription Medications?	No

Increased Risks

Indicator	Value

Health Problems of Greatest Importance to Patient

Constant aching back.
Tired all the time.
Can't move my bowels.

RESOURCE 2B: CARE GUIDE TARGETS AND RED FLAGS

Condition	Targets	Red Flags
General	Adherence to medications	Almost out of any medication
Constipation	Three soft stools per week Minimal straining Minimal bloating	Abdominal pain Nausea and vomiting Rectal bleeding
Depression	Depression does not limit ability to do desired activities.	↑ symptoms ↑ use of alcohol Suicidal thoughts
Osteoarthritis	OA pain does not limit ability to do desired activities.	↑ pain
Persistent pain	Pain does not limit ability to do desired activities.	↑ pain New/increased confusion Falls

RESOURCE 2B: CARE GUIDE TARGETS AND RED FLAGS *(Continued)*

Constipation

Current Care Guide

Diet

32+ oz of oral fluid intake daily

High-fiber diet: bran, fruits, vegetables

Education

Discuss the range of "normal" bowel function

Medications

Judicious, step-care use of laxatives: fiber/bulk, stimulant, osmotic, enema

Minimize use of constipating medications: opiates, iron, diuretics, antacids, Ca-blockers, anti-cholinergics, anti-histamines, anti-psychotics, cholestyramine, clonidine

Monitoring

PCP office visits every 3 months

Pt to call GCN every month

Targets

Minimal bloating

Minimal straining

Soft stools per week = 3

Red Flags

Abdominal pain

Nausea and vomiting

Rectal bleeding

Background Information

Year of onset	2003
Straining occurrences per week	7
Incomplete evacuations per week	2
Abdominal bloating occurrences per week	7
# of BMs per week	2
Typical consistency	Hard

Current Management

Daily oral hydration	32+ oz

Most Recent Results

Measure	Date	Results

(Continued)

RESOURCE 2B: CARE GUIDE TARGETS AND RED FLAGS *(Continued)*

Depression

Current Care Guide

Medications

SSRI: sertaline (Zoloft), paroxetine (Paxil), citalopram (Celexa), escitalopram (Lexapro)

Monitoring

PCP office visits every 3 months

Pt to call GCN every month

Regular visits with mental health professional

Other

Remove exposure to contributing factors: medications, alcohol

Targets

Depression limits the ability to do desired activities = No

Red Flags

Increased symptoms of depression

Increased use of alcohol

Suicidal ideation

Background Information

Year of onset	1998
History of depression	Yes
Suicidal activity	No
Recent losses or crises	No

Previous Management

Medicine	depression meds
Medicine - reason for stopping or not starting	sick to stomach

Most Recent Results

Measure	Date	Results
Alcohol use (drinks/week)	7/2008	0

RESOURCE 2B: CARE GUIDE TARGETS AND
RED FLAGS *(Continued)*

Disability

Current Care Guide

Monitoring

PCP office visits every 3 months

Pt to call GCN every month

Targets

Red Flags

Persistently increased pain

Background Information

Year of onset	0000
Physical barrier to home entry	stairs to 2nd floor ap
Physical barrier inside home	none
Resource used to manage transportation/walking outside home	Person
Resource used to manage shopping	Person
Resource used to manage light housework	Person
Resource used to manage bathing	Person
Unsafe stove	no

Most Recent Results

Measure	Date	Results

(Continued)

RESOURCE 2B: CARE GUIDE TARGETS AND RED FLAGS *(Continued)*

Osteoarthritis

Current Care Guide

Medication

For chronic pain: acetaminophen 650-1000 mg po TID-QID

For exacerbations of pain: Add NSAID and/or capsaicin cream temporarily. Avoid NSAID in PUD, CHF,HTN, and renal insufficiency

If acetaminophen, NSAID, and capsaicin not effective, add an opiod temporarily. Observe for adverseeffects of opioids: cognition, constipation

Monitoring

PCP office visits every 3 month

Pt to call GCN every month

Physical Activity

Regular mild-moderate exercise for flexibility, strength, and/or endurance

Referral

Education and counselin

Targets

Pain limits person's ability to do desired activities = No

Red Flags

Background Information

Year of onset	1991
Area(s) most affected	Hip, Knee, Spine
Functional limitation by arthritis	A lot

Previous Management

Medicine	Vioxx
Medicine - reason for stopping or not starting	dangerous

Most Recent Results

Measure	Date	Results
BUN	2/2006	30
Creatinine	2/2006	1.5
X-ray - Joint/Bon	2/2007	normal

RESOURCE 2B: CARE GUIDE TARGETS AND RED FLAGS *(Continued)*

Persistent Pain

Current Care Guide

Education

Encourage pain education, self-management, and cognitive-behavioral therapy

Medications

Acetaminophen (e.g., Tylenol) 650-1000 mg po TID-QID. Do not exceed 4g per 24 hrs. Reduce dose 50-7 in liver disease or alcoholism.

Avoid: propoxyphere (Darvon), tramadol (Ultram), methadone (Dolophine)

For exacerbations of pain: Add NSAID and/or capsaicin cream temporarily. Avoid NSAID in PUD, CHF, HTN, and renal insufficiency.

If Acetaminophen is not effective, add a non-acetylated salicylate: salsalate (e.g., Disalcid), trisalicylate (e.g., Trilisate)

If an opioid is not effective, add an adjuvant: nortriptyline (e.g., Aventil) if patient is depressed, or carbamazepine (Tegretol) if pain is neuropathic.

If non-acetylated salicylate is not effective, add an opioid: oxycodone (OxyContin), morphine (MSContin) transdermal fentanyl (Duragesic).

If taking an opioid, protect against and monitor for serious adverse side effects: constipation, impairment in cognition (car crash), gait, balance (falls).

Monitoring

Maintain a record of pain level daily

PCP office visits every 3 months

Pt to call GCN every month

Other

Treat underlying cause of pain, if possible

Targets

Pain limits person's ability to do desired activities = No

Red Flags

Confusion

Constipation

Falls

Persistently increased pain

Background Information

Year of onset	1998
Description	Aching
Most affected	Hip, Knee, Back
Cause	Arthritis
Pain limits	Daily activities, social activities, Quality of life

Current Management

Physical Treatments	Heat, salve

(Continued)

RESOURCE 2B: CARE GUIDE TARGETS AND RED FLAGS *(Continued)*

Previous Management

Medicine	pain meds
Medicine - reason for stopping or not starting	causes constipation

Most Recent Results

Measure	Date	Results
ALT	2/2006	44
AST	2/2006	50

RESOURCE 2C: ACTION PLAN

°°°NOTIFY EILEEN IF I GO TO THE HOSPITAL!!!!!°°°

My Action Plan

Guided Care Nurse:	**Eileen Novak, RN: 202-816-6798**
Primary Physician:	Dr. Benchaim, MD: 202-891-4233
Pharmacy:Rite Aid:	202-399-6688

Morning	Noon	Afternoon	Bedtime

Take these medications, even if I feel great: Notes

	Morning	Noon	Afternoon	Bedtime	Notes
Sertraline				1 pill	For my mood
Nabumetone	3 pills	3 pills			For joint pain
Acetaminophen	1 pill	1 pill			For joint pain
Metamucil	1 teaspoon				For constipation

Medicine
Order refills before running out of medications
Inform Eileen of any medication changes
Only take medicine prescribed to me

Diet
Drink four glasses of water every day.
Eat more fruits and vegetables.

My Personal health goals:

Physical Activity
Walk 10 minutes, three days per week.
Practice light stretching in the morning.

1. **Reduce my back pain**
2. **Have more energy**

(Continued)

RESOURCE 2C: ACTION PLAN *(Continued)*

Check Myself	Target	Red Flag
Keep daily pain journal	Do all my daily activities	More pain, falling, confusion
Keep track of my mood		More depression, feeling hopeless

Check-Ups
Call my Guided Care nurse first Tuesday every month
Regular checkup with Dr. Benchaim every three months
September 5–Oct. 10, Wednesdays, 10 a.m.–12:30 p.m.

Specialists
See physical therapist every Friday morning
CDSM class at Glendale Baptist Church,

Preventing Problems
Get flu shot in the fall
Screening schedule Nov. 1, 2009, 10 a.m., Washington Hospital Center

Other
Bring Action Plan to all appointments with medical professionals.

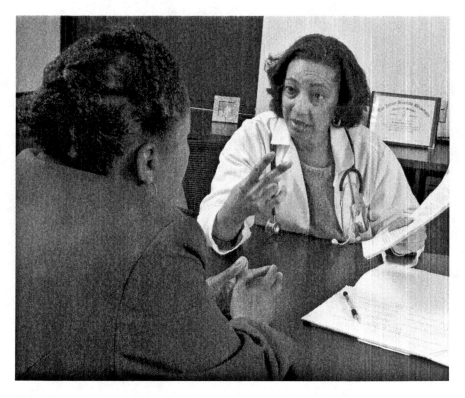

Photo 3.1 A primary care physician and a Guided Care nurse meeting to personalize a patient's Preliminary Care Guide.

CREDIT: Photo by Larry Canner.

3 Is Your Practice Ready to Adopt Guided Care?

Primary care practices in the United States are struggling. Reimbursement for their care of chronically ill patients is inadequate. Science and technology are advancing; as a result, methods of care are proliferating. Practitioners are expected to incorporate new practice guidelines into every patient encounter despite shrinking visit times and expanding requirements for care documentation. Interoperative health information technology is needed to support care coordination and clinical decision making, but the cost of incorporating it is a major barrier to most practices. Premiums for liability insurance are high, and the risk of lawsuits is ever-present. Medical students' debt loads are heavy, and primary care incomes are low. No wonder fewer American medical students and residents are choosing careers in primary care and geriatrics! To make matters worse, the United States also has a serious and growing shortage of registered nurses. As the nation's population is aging, its workforce for providing chronic care is becoming increasingly overwhelmed.

These challenges are daunting, but recent trends offer hope that rejuvenated primary care practices may flourish in the years ahead. Our national leaders—and the public—are becoming increasingly aware of the growing need for chronic care that is both comprehensive and well coordinated. In fact, during his 2008 campaign for President of the United States, Barack Obama touted care coordination by medical

53

homes as a high-priority goal. The Institute of Medicine's 2008 report, "Retooling for an Aging America: Building the Health Care Workforce," asserts that "the Medicare system will need to be flexible in paying for innovative models of care. Interdisciplinary models that support collaboration among multiple types of providers will be essential in improving care delivery for older adults" (Rowe et al., 2008).

Reaching these goals will require more than rhetoric; our leaders and practitioners will need to make difficult decisions, readjust operational and funding priorities, and implement new forms of primary care practice. The first step in this new direction is the national Medicare Medical Home Demonstration (MMHD), which the Centers for Medicare & Medicaid Services (CMS) plans to launch in 2009. Several other tests of the medical home concept are in various stages of development as variations of the medical home are being pilot tested by employers, private insurers, and state Medicaid programs.

During the MMHD, approximately 400 practices in eight states will receive supplemental care management payments in return for providing several essential chronic care services to their patients who have chronic health conditions. In each such medical home, the physician caring for chronically ill Medicare beneficiaries must:

- Advocate for and provide ongoing support, oversight and guidance in implementing a care plan that provides integrated, coherent, cross-disciplinary care in partnership with the beneficiary and all other physicians furnishing care to the beneficiary.
- Use evidence-based medicine and evidence-based clinical support tools to guide decision making at the point of care.
- Use health information technology (HIT) that may include remote monitoring and patient registries to monitor and track the health status of beneficiaries.
- Provide Medicare beneficiaries with enhanced and convenient access to health care.

Practices that do not routinely provide these services to their chronically ill patients could use CMS's supplemental payments to provide them by implementing an electronic health record and by:

- Outsourcing required services (e.g., contracting with disease management companies),
- Enhancing the ability of its current physicians and staff to provide these services, or

- Expanding the practice's personnel (e.g., adopting the Guided Care model).

The goal of this chapter is to help practices determine their readiness to rejuvenate the chronic care they provide by adopting the Guided Care model and participating in either the MMHD or other demonstrations of the medical home. The following sections outline some of the benefits, requirements, and logistics of adopting the Guided Care model and participating in a demonstration of the medical home.

THE BENEFITS TO PRACTICES THAT ADOPT GUIDED CARE

Would the adoption of Guided Care benefit our patients? Would it benefit the people who work in our practice? These are important questions for a practice to answer in considering whether to adopt Guided Care. In this section, we provide brief summaries of the available information about the effects of Guided Care on patients and their health care providers. This evidence is derived from a pilot study ($n = 150$) and a multi-center, randomized controlled trial ($n = 904$) of Guided Care conducted by Johns Hopkins University in eight urban and suburban primary care practices in communities in the mid-Atlantic United States between 2003 and 2007 (Boult, Reider, et al., 2008; Boyd et al., 2008; Leff et al., 2008; Sylvia et al., 2008).

Effects of Guided Care on Patients

In both the pilot test and the randomized trial, patients who received Guided Care rated the quality of their health care more highly than did similar patients who received "usual care." In fact, in the randomized trial, those who received Guided Care were twice as likely to rate the quality of their care in the highest category (see Table 2.4, p. 25). All of the study participants rated their care on the validated, 20-item "patient assessment of chronic illness care" (PACIC) instrument during telephone interviews with professional interviewers who did not know whether the participants were receiving Guided Care or usual care. The items included in the PACIC address providers' communication, coordination of care, and knowledge of the patient, which are at least as important indicators of quality of care for multimorbid patients as providers' diagnostic, screening, or therapeutic activities.

Anecdotally, most patients and caregivers express high levels of appreciation for and satisfaction with Guided Care (see interviews at www. guidedcare.org). They particularly value the easy access to medical advice and the security and peace of mind that comes from having a health care professional who knows their health and social circumstances very well. Many patients and caregivers have commented, "It's like having a nurse in the family."

Effects of Guided Care on Physicians

The 49 physicians who participated in the randomized trial of Guided Care were surveyed anonymously at baseline and 1 year after the study began. Compared to the physicians who continued to provide usual care, the physicians who worked with a Guided Care nurse for a year reported greater increases in satisfaction with communication with patients and family caregivers, with education of family caregivers, with motivation of patients to care for themselves, and with knowing patients' medications (see Table 2.3, p. 24).

Anecdotally, before the study, most of the participating physicians expressed skepticism about working with a Guided Care nurse. A year later, 23 of the 25 physicians who had worked with a Guided Care nurse said they had benefited from working with the nurse, and all 25 chose to continue working with the nurse for an optional additional year. To the extent that Guided Care increases physicians' satisfaction with the care of some of their most challenging patients, it may also enhance professional pride and, thereby, recruitment and retention of physicians in primary care practices.

Effects of Guided Care on Practice Revenue

The traditional fee-for-service Medicare program does not reimburse practices for many of the costs of providing Guided Care, for example, the nurse's salary and benefits, electronic equipment, health information technology, and travel. During its MMHD, however, CMS will pay care management fees to participating practices, in addition to the standard fee-for-service payments, to cover the practices' costs for providing specified medical home services to Medicare beneficiaries with chronic conditions. Guided Care is one approach that practices may adopt for providing many of these specified services.

At the time this book went to press, CMS had proposed to pay per-patient care management fees that would be higher for Tier 2 practices and higher for high-risk Medicare beneficiaries. For a physician with a panel of 1,400 patients, 20% of whom are Medicare beneficiaries, these fees would average approximately $149,000 per year (see Appendix D: CMS's Medicare Medical Home Demonstration, Table D.2). The amounts of the care management fees that participating physicians will actually receive must be approved by the federal Office of Management and Budget; its decision was expected in early 2009.

The law that mandated CMS to conduct the MMHD also requires that participating practices receive "shared savings." That is, 80% of the net savings realized by the Medicare program as a result of the demonstration must also be paid to the participating practices. During a pilot test (Sylvia et al., 2008) and the early months of a randomized trial (Leff et al., 2008), Guided Care reduced insurers' expenditures by 10% to 20%. Although less certain, shared savings payments may provide additional revenue to the practices participating in the MMHD.

As discussed in chapter 7, the costs of providing Guided Care must be weighed against these additional revenues. Nevertheless, providing Guided Care services and meeting CMS's other requirements for participating in the MMHD (see Appendix D) would substantially increase a practice's annual revenues. Further, if the MMHD is successful, CMS may continue to offer supplemental payments to practices that provide medical home services for Medicare beneficiaries with chronic health conditions after the demonstration is completed in 2012.

REQUIREMENTS FOR ADOPTING GUIDED CARE

Practices that are interested in obtaining the benefits of Guided Care need to determine whether they can meet four requirements.

Sufficient Number of Patients With Chronic Conditions

The typical caseload of a Guided Care nurse is 50 to 60 patients, each of whom has several chronic health conditions (see Table 3.1). The practice must have a total panel of patients that is large enough that it contains enough chronically ill patients to constitute a caseload for the nurse. For example, a typical practice that has a panel of about 1,500 adult patients provides ongoing care for about 300 patients who are age 65 years or

Table 3.1

CHARACTERISTICS OF GUIDED CARE PATIENTS

	TOTAL ($N = 904$)	GUIDED CARE ($N = 485$)	USUAL CARE ($N = 419$)
SOCIODEMOGRAPHIC FACTORS			
Age, mean years (range)	77.7 (66–106)	77.2 (66–106)	78.1 (66–96)
Sex (percentage female)	54.8	54.2	55.4
Race (percentage)			
White	50.0	51.1	48.9
Black	46.0	45.6	46.3
Other	4.0	3.3	4.8
Ethnicity (percentage Hispanic)	1.7	1.9	1.4
Marital status (percentage)			
Married	47.3	46.0	48.5
Divorced/separated	11.2	11.6	10.7
Widowed	37.5	37.9	37.0
Never married	4.0	4.5	3.8
Education (percentage 12+ years)	45.0	46.4	43.4
Finances at end of month (percentage)			
Some money left over	54.5	57.9	51.1
Just enough money left over	33.5	32.8	34.2
Not enough money left over	12.0	9.3	14.7
Habitation status (percentage living alone)	31.3	32.0	30.6
Type of Medicare (percentage)			
HMO-A	44.8	42.1	47.5
Fee-for-service	34.1	31. 7	36.5
HMO-B	21.1	26. 2	16.0

(Continued)

Table 3.1

CHARACTERISTICS OF GUIDED CARE PATIENTS *(Continued)*

	TOTAL (N = 904)	GUIDED CARE (N = 485)	USUAL CARE (N = 419)
HEALTH AND FUNCTIONAL STATUS			
Hierarchical condition category (HCC) score,[a] mean	2.1	2.1	2.0
Self-rated health, mean			
Excellent	2.8	2.5	3.1
Very good	16.8	20.0	13.6
Good	37.1	37.7	36.5
Fair	31.2	30.1	32.2
Poor	12.2	9.7	14.6
Mean number of self-reported conditions, mean (range)	4.3 (0–13)	4.3 (0–13)	4.3 (0–12)
Difficulty with 1+ ADL[b] (percentage)	30.1	30.9	29.3
Difficulty with 2+ IADL[c] (percentage)	23.6	19.6	27.6
Receives help from a person (percentage)	50.1	45.2	54.9
Short Form-36 score, mean (range)			
Physical component summary	38.4 (6.7–63.1)	38.7 (13.8–63.0)	38.1 (6.7–63.1)
Mental component summary	49.5 (6.4–71.9)	50.3 (6.4–70.0)	48.7 (13.7–71.9)
Short portable mental status mean (range)	9.1 (3–10)	9.1 (4–10)	9.0 (3–10)

[a]Hierarchical condition category (HCC) scores indicate the likelihood that Medicare beneficiaries, based on their medical conditions, will use health care services heavily during the coming year. An HCC score of 1.0 indicates that a person has average risk. An HCC score of 2.0 indicates twice the average risk. [b]ADL = activities of daily living. [c]IADL = instrumental activities of daily living.

older. On average, about 60 to 75 (20% to 25%) of these patients have several chronic health conditions. Practices with larger panels may be able to support more than one Guided Care nurse. A Guided Care nurse could be shared if two smaller practices were in close proximity to each other.

Office Space

The Guided Care nurse operates most effectively in a secure, quiet office that is located near the physicians' offices and is sufficiently private for communication with patients and their caregivers by telephone. This office should provide the nurse with broadband Internet access and convenient access to the practice's staff, medical records, supplies, and office equipment.

Health Information Technology

As described in the preceding chapter, several clinical activities of a Guided Care nurse are supported by health information technology. A practice that already has such technology might need to upgrade its system to support the activities of the Guided Care nurse. A practice that does not have health information technology would need to acquire a locally installed or web-based system that supports the activities of Guided Care. At the time this book went to press, several commercial vendors provided health information technology to support the activities of Guided Care and the medical home. Up-to-the-moment information about the capabilities and availability of these products is available at www.centerforhit.org; www.transforMED.org/MedicalHomeMarketplace and www.acponline.org. Additional details about required health information technology are provided in the next chapter and in Appendix D.

Commitment of Physicians and Staff

The integration of a new type of health care provider into a primary care practice is a process that requires careful planning, optimism, open communication, honest feedback, flexibility, perseverance, and patience. It is important that all members of the practice are committed to making the process successful, as occasional obstacles and setbacks are inevitable. As discussed in greater detail in chapter 5, the successful integration of a Guided Care nurse into a primary care practice proceeds through several steps:

- Orient the nurse to the roles, responsibilities, and priorities of the physicians and all the members of the office staff, including the practice's routine operation and flow.
- Orient the physicians and office staff to the roles, responsibilities, and priorities of the nurse.
- Achieve consensus among the nurse, the physicians, and the office staff about the optimal approaches to working as a team, acknowledging existing lines of authority and accountability.
- Develop plans for monitoring and managing the nurse.
- Discuss the process by which patients are selected to receive Guided Care with all members of the office team.
- Orient the nurse to the supportive and health-related resources in the local community (e.g., hospitals, skilled nursing facilities, home care agencies, rehabilitation facilities, the Area Agency on Aging, Meals on Wheels, senior centers, and adult day health care centers).
- If the practice will participate in the MMHD, orient its physicians and staff to the additional structures and functions required for recognition as a medical home (details in Appendix D).

PARTICIPATING IN A MEDICAL HOME DEMONSTRATION

Practices that desire the benefits of Guided Care and can meet the preceding requirements will probably need to participate in a demonstration of the medical home to obtain the supplemental revenues necessary to cover the costs of providing Guided Care. Several such demonstrations are in various stages of development in different regions of the United States (see Appendix D within "A Purchaser's Guide for the Patient-Centered Medical Home" at www.pcpcc.net/content/purchaser-guide for current information). The largest is CMS's national MMHD. To participate, practices will need to apply and show that they can provide the required medical home services (see the detailed discussion of the MMHD in Appendix D). According to the plans in effect when this book went to press, CMS intended to:

- Issue invitations in January 2009 for applications for the MMHD from hundreds of practices in eight states.
- Evaluate practices' applications and capabilities throughout the remainder of 2009.

- Begin paying care management fees to participating practices in January 2010.

Beginning in mid-2009, the Centers for Medicare & Medicaid Services will provide practices with high-level guidance in completing a self-attestation survey and submitting documentation of their capabilities for providing medical home services. This guidance may include biweekly training sessions conducted by conference calls and Web-based seminars.

Assistance in meeting the qualifications for recognition as a medical home will be provided by the Roger C. Lipitz Center for Integrated Health Care at the Johns Hopkins Bloomberg School of Public Health and several partner organizations. As detailed in chapter 7, this assistance will include an online course for physicians, an online course for registered nurses, information about the capabilities of commercially available electronic health records, regional in-person workshops, information by telephone and Internet, and on-site consultation.

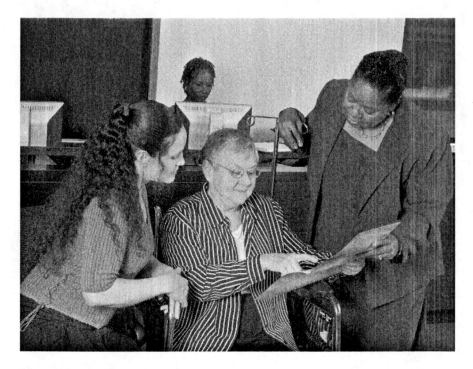

Photo 4.1 A Guided Care nurse discussing a Preliminary Care Guide with a patient and a family caregiver.

CREDIT: Photo by Larry Canner.

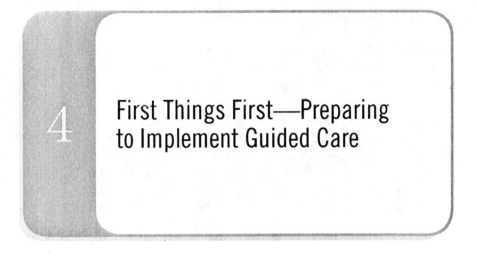

First Things First—Preparing to Implement Guided Care

4

Transforming a medical practice into a full medical home is an ambitious undertaking. To implement the necessary changes requires courage, creativity, leadership, flexibility, and perseverance, but most who have done it are pleased with their transformed practices.

Leaders who set out to make this transformation must choose wisely among several operational strategies and tactics, including (a) outsourcing chronic care services; (b) retraining and redeploying their present staff; or (c) redesigning their practice to include new providers, new roles, and new tools.

This chapter describes how a practice can acquire many of the capabilities of a medical home by adopting the Guided Care model. A detailed description of all the requirements for recognition as a medical home is provided in Appendix D: CMS's Medicare Medical Home Demonstration. Here we focus on describing many of the operational steps involved in preparing a practice—large or small—to transform its chronic care abilities through Guided Care. Based on 5 years of practical experience in testing Guided Care in primary care practices, this chapter provides detailed information about preparing the practice's personnel (i.e., physicians and other staff), patients, and infrastructure (i.e., physical space and information technology). Finally, it offers advice on selecting and hiring a Guided Care nurse.

IDENTIFYING FINANCIAL RESOURCES

In today's challenging economy, sustainable transformation of medical practices to provide excellent chronic care requires both an *initial* investment of resources to make the necessary changes in the practice and an *adequate* source of revenue to support the ongoing operation of the new care model. In most cases, the investment of resources for the initial transformation must be made by the practice or its parent organization. Few public or private insurers will provide substantial financial support to alter private practices or health care delivery systems.

The magnitude of the initial investment needed to prepare a practice to provide Guided Care is variable, but modest. Essential resources, to be described in greater detail later in this chapter, include:

- *Time* to orient the practice's physicians and office staff to the roles and responsibilities of the Guided Care nurse, and to their new roles and responsibilities in collaborating with the Guided Care nurse in caring for patients with multiple chronic conditions. These few hours may be more than recovered through the increases in practice efficiency produced by Guided Care.
- *Space* in the office for the Guided Care nurse.
- *Equipment* needed by the Guided Care nurse (i.e., a laptop computer, a cellular telephone, and access to the Internet).
- *Information technology* to support the clinical activities of Guided Care.

A prerequisite for a practice to make such initial investments in transformation is the assurance that the transformed practice will subsequently generate new supplemental revenue and/or realize cost savings that will support its operation. Fortunately, public and private health care insurers are increasingly accepting responsibility for providing such supplemental revenue. As illustrated in Figure 4.1, some insurers are paying management fees to transformed practices as investments in efficient, high-quality chronic care. This prevents health crises and, thereby, averts the need for more expensive care in hospitals, emergency departments, and skilled nursing facilities, ultimately reducing the insurer's expenditures.

A tangible example of the availability of revenue that would support transformed chronic care is the "care management" fee that the

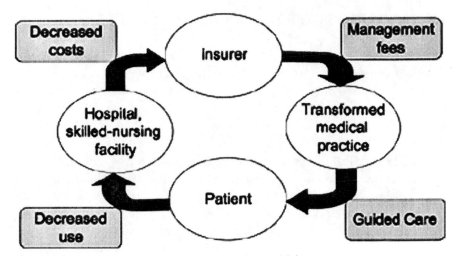

Figure 4.1 Allocation of resources for Guided Care model.

Centers for Medicare & Medicaid Services (CMS) will pay to practices that participate in its national Medicare Medical Home Demonstration (MMHD) beginning in 2010. Other private and public insurers and self-insured employers are also paying supplemental fees to practices to support other demonstrations of transformed chronic care (see Appendix D within "A Purchaser's Guide for the Patient-Centered Medical Home" at www.pcpcc.net/content/purchaser-guide). Because Guided Care provides many of the core services that define the medical home, a Guided Care practice could apply to participate in one of these demonstrations of the medical home and, thereby, obtain the supplemental revenue needed to support its operation. If the results of these demonstrations are favorable, the involved insurers are likely to continue to offer supplemental care management fees in return for efficient, effective chronic care.

In summary, practices preparing to implement the Guided Care model will probably need to identify internal resources to support some of the necessary initial changes in the practice, for example, the orientation of patients and personnel, and the procurement of the needed space, equipment, and information technology. Such practices will also need to enter into contracts with insurers that will provide ongoing payments to support high-quality chronic care, such as the care management fees being offered to participants in the ongoing medical home demonstrations.

PREPARING THE PHYSICIANS AND OFFICE STAFF

As noted in chapter 3, introducing a new health care professional, in this case a registered nurse, into an established practice requires careful planning, detailed orientation of the existing staff, and ample opportunities for discussion in order to create an effective new team. Some initial confusion and resistance should be anticipated and addressed. Change theory specifies that an appropriate champion for transformation, for example, a medical director or practice administrator who demonstrates commitment and leadership throughout the process, is essential to a successful practice transformation.

All physicians and staff members within the practice should receive clear, compelling information about the practice's goals and reasons for adopting Guided Care. They should also receive detailed descriptions of how Guided Care operates and how they will need to adjust some established roles and procedures to collaborate effectively with the Guided Care nurse. As described in chapter 7 and referenced in Appendix A: Online Courses, physicians may take a formal online course designed to help them function effectively in medical homes (see www.medhomeinfo.org for more information).

Because the Guided Care nurse has a unique and novel role in the practice, the nurse's smooth integration into the existing office personnel is aided by ensuring that these employees understand the scope of the work of a Guided Care nurse, how patients are selected to receive Guided Care, and why the Guided Care nurse is restricted to providing only certain clinical services to only selected patients. The distribution of written descriptive materials helps to ensure that everyone obtains and can refer back to the same information. Such materials include brief descriptions of the nurse's role and responsibilities (Boyd et al., 2007) and the physician's role and responsibilities (see Table 4.1).

Each physician leads a practice team, including the nurse, that cares for a panel of patients. As outlined in Tables 4.1 and 6.1, the physician is responsible for communicating regularly with the nurse about their patients and their teamwork. The physician is also involved in hiring, orienting, and evaluating the nurse. The nurse, may be a member of several such teams, one for each physician in the practice.

As described more fully in chapter 7, extensive technical assistance for the adoption of Guided Care and for the transition of a practice to

Table 4.1

THE PHYSICIAN'S ROLE AND RESPONSIBILITIES IN GUIDED CARE

Nurse selection	Each physician with whom the nurse will work should review resumes, conduct interviews, and participate in the ranking of applicants.
Nurse orientation	As described in chapter 5, each physician should meet with the nurse several times during the nurse's orientation to define how they will work together to care for patients. The physicians should also introduce Guided Care patients to the nurse during routine office visits and allow the nurse to observe the physician's style of interacting with these patients and their caregivers.
Building the caseload	The physician meets with the nurse for 20 to 25 minutes per patient to discuss and revise the Preliminary Care Guide that the nurse creates following the initial home assessment.
Ongoing Guided Care	The physician notifies the nurse of changes in their mutual patients' clinical status, especially admission to hospitals and emergency departments and referrals to specialists. The physician also replies to the nurse's messages about their patients' clinical conditions. To optimize their working relationship, the physician and the nurse meet periodically to give each other feedback and to refine their patterns of communication and collaboration. The physician also participates in the practice's periodic evaluation of the nurse's performance.

one that meets the criteria for recognition as a medical home is available to leaders of practices and their parent organizations. For those who are interested in participating in the MMHD, free advice is available by telephone, and valuable practice self-assessment tools and information about health information technology are accessible by visiting www.medhomeinfo.org. On-site consultation and implementation workshops are available at market rates.

After all of the practice's physicians and staff members have received this information, they should be given ample opportunity to ask questions, discuss their thoughts with the medical director and/or practice administrator, and help plan the details of implementing Guided Care. A discussion outline resembling the one that follows may help maximize the value of such conversations during staff meetings.

DISCUSSION: INTEGRATING GUIDED CARE INTO THE PRACTICE

- Guided Care introduction (given by the medical director and/or practice administrator).
  - Inform attendees that the practice has committed to adopting Guided Care.
  - Explain the practice's rationale for adopting Guided Care.
  - Acknowledge that change is difficult and slow, but highlight the benefits of such change in the long run.
  - Confirm that attendees have received a written description of Guided Care.
- Describe how Guided Care will work in the practice.
  - Sources of funding.
  - Plans for: hiring the nurse(s), identifying eligible patients, communicating with patients, equipping office space.
  - Plans for: orienting the nurse, holding nurse–staff meetings.
- Questions and discussion.

PREPARING PATIENTS AND THEIR CAREGIVERS

Patients with multiple chronic conditions (and their family caregivers) have experienced firsthand the fragmentation, inefficiency, and frustration associated with contemporary chronic care. Most of them would quickly recognize and appreciate the value of having access to a health care professional who knows them personally, encourages them, monitors them, coordinates their care, and connects them with needed services. Most, however, are not yet aware of Guided Care. Some may confuse it with more familiar programs such as care management and disease management. Therefore, each practice that decides to adopt Guided Care should conduct a campaign to inform its patients and their family caregivers of the new care model and to make it clear that it will be offered only to those whom their insurer approves.

To be most effective, this informational campaign should be multifaceted and timed to coincide with the Guided Care nurse's arrival in the practice. Clear, concise, consistent, and accurate messages communicated through several channels are most likely to succeed. Personalized versions of resource 4A: Letter to Patients Describing Guided Care at the end of this chapter could be mailed to the patients and also posted on the practice's Web site, if applicable. Posters like Resource 4B: Guided Care Waiting Room Poster could be hung in the waiting room. Physicians and members of the office staff should be prepared to give knowledgeable verbal endorsement and to answer patients' and caregivers' questions about Guided Care to further reinforce the effectiveness of this campaign.

IDENTIFYING PATIENTS WHO ARE ELIGIBLE TO RECEIVE GUIDED CARE SERVICES

Since the supplemental revenue for each eligible patient, which allows the practice to afford Guided Care, comes from patients' health insurers, the criteria for patients' eligibility to receive Guided Care are usually set by insurers.

For example, for practices that participate in the MMHD, CMS will identify, from its enrollment and claims files, all of a practice's patients who may be eligible for the demonstration. As explained in greater detail in Appendix D, these eligibility criteria include:

- Being enrolled in Medicare Part A.
- Being enrolled in Medicare Part B.
- Not being enrolled in Medicare's hospice, end stage renal disease, or Medicare Advantage programs.
- Not being a long-term resident in a nursing home.
- Having at least one qualifying chronic disease (a list of qualifying diseases is provided in Appendix D, Resource D.1).
- Receiving the bulk of their recent primary care from the practice.

As patients are identified as eligible to receive Guided Care, they should be notified of their eligibility, and their names and contact information should be given to the Guided Care nurse and the patient's physicians. If the practice is participating in the MMHD, eligible patients will then need to sign a voluntary agreement to receive medical home services (and to generate care management fees) through one specific personal physician in the practice, usually their established primary care physician. As described in the next chapter, this begins the process of establishing Guided Care for these patients. Once established, Guided Care usually continues for the remainder of these patients' lives.

Designating Office Space for the Nurse(s)

One of the most important processes underlying the success of Guided Care is effective teamwork among the Guided Care nurse and the practice's physicians and other staff members. As discussed in subsequent chapters, several factors promote teamwork, not the least of which is working in contiguous space that facilitates frequent and easy communication with coworkers. Thus, the practice should designate an office located near the physicians' offices and the work areas of the other staff members for the Guided Care nurse.

The nurse's office should be a functional, private work space that accommodates a laptop computer, file cabinets, and broadband access to the Internet. This office should be sufficiently private to allow the nurse to store confidential medical information and to conduct frequent personal conversations by telephone (and occasionally in person) with patients and their caregivers. It must also provide the nurse with convenient access to the practice's staff, medical records, supplies, and office equipment.

Health Information Technology

Many of the clinical activities of Guided Care are supported by health information technology (HIT). For example:

- After completing a detailed initial assessment of a new Guided Care patient, the nurse enters the patient's diagnoses and all other assessment information into the HIT.
- The diagnoses evoke preloaded evidence-based guidelines for managing each of the patient's chronic conditions.
- The HIT integrates the guidelines for all of the patient's conditions into the Preliminary Care Guide (Resource 2A), and it checks for and reports possible serious adverse interactions among the patient's medications.
- The nurse enters reminders to perform specific clinical actions for individual patients on specific dates in the future. Each day, the

HIT displays a list of the actions that are due to be completed that day.

- The Guided Care nurse documents all encounters with patients, caregivers, and health care professionals in the HIT.
- The practice's administrator—or medical director, in small practices—queries the HIT to track documented nurse–patient encounters and the nurse's adherence to preestablished standards for frequency and content of encounters with patients.

For practices that do not already use HIT, there are two options for obtaining the necessary technology. The first is to license access to Web-based software that supports Guided Care. The second is to install and maintain similar software on a local server. Practices that already use HIT may need to enhance it by activating or adding new features that allow the system to support the core functions of Guided Care. Specific information about the capabilities and prices of a wide variety of electronic health records for medical offices is available at www.centerforhit. org and www.acponline.org.

Selecting a Guided Care Nurse

The most important decision in preparing to provide Guided Care is the selection of the right Guided Care nurse. This employee will have important relationships with the physicians, the other office staff members, and many of the sickest patients in the practice. Turnover in such positions is disruptive and expensive, so conducting a careful search is worth the required time and effort. The minimum requirements for applicants are:

- Current licensure as a registered nurse.
- Completion of an accredited online course in Guided Care nursing (available at www.ijhn.jhmi.edu/calendar.asp). The course outline is shown in Appendix A. Tuition is free for nurses employed by practices participating in the MMHD. This course could be completed between a nurse's hiring and starting to work in a Guided Care practice.
- A Certificate in Guided Care Nursing issued by the American Nurses Credentialing Center. The Certificate could be earned between a nurse's hiring and starting to work in a Guided Care practice.

- A minimum of 3 years of nursing experience, preferably with older patients.
- Skill in using computers, the Internet, and health information technology.
- Ability to travel frequently to hospitals, skilled nursing facilities, patients' homes, and other sites where patients receive care (as indicated by patients' needs).

Highly desirable qualities include:

- Excellent interpersonal skills.
- Flexible and creative problem-solving skills.
- Good clinical judgment and decision-making skills.
- Demonstrated ability to work effectively as a member of an interdisciplinary team.
- Demonstrated ability to work independently.
- Clear understanding of the role of Guided Care nurse.
- Desire to learn and practice all of the position's components.
- Commitment to "coaching" (rather than "teaching") patients to improve their health behaviors to attain their health-related goals.
- Commitment to learning about and referring patients to health-related services in the local community.
- Effective oral and written communication skills.
- Effective listening and assertion skills.

To identify candidates for the position of Guided Care nurse, versions of the job descriptions and advertisements shown at the end of this chapter, Resource 4C: Job Description and Resource 4D: Sample Advertisement for Guided Care Nurse, respectively, may be submitted to local newspapers, nursing journals, newsletters, and local chapters of national health professional societies, such as the Case Management Society of America and the National Gerontological Nurses Association.

Median salary levels for nurse care managers vary considerably depending on the nurse's experience and certification and the geographical region of the United States where the position is offered (Case Management Society of America, 2005). To attract good applicants, the practice should offer a salary that is competitive with local hospital and home health care employers. Qualified applicants should receive a detailed written description of the position before their interviews, and they should discuss the many components of the position thoroughly during their interviews.

Because of the importance of hiring a Guided Care nurse who will be compatible with the particular practice, it is useful to conduct interviews and ratings of qualified applicants by the practice's administrator, medical director, physicians and any other providers. A scale for rating applicants is shown in Table 4.2. Discrepancies among ratings should be resolved by conversations among the raters and, sometimes, by conducting supplemental interviews.

The importance of hiring the right nurse cannot be overstated. Therefore, if none of the initial applicants is acceptable, another round of advertising and interviewing should be conducted. To allow sufficient time for the placement of advertisements, the completion of multiple

Table 4.2

GUIDED CARE NURSE APPLICANT RATING SCALE

	Applicants	
Qualification	Eileen Novak	Susan Weber
1. Affinity for multimorbid seniors	5	3
2. Experience in hospital and community	4	5
3. Affinity for coaching	5	2
4. Flexibility in problem solving	2	4
5. Comfort working with physicians	3	3
6. Organized work style	4	5
7. Communication skills	4	2
8. Experience with information technology	5	2
9. Assertiveness	4	5
10. Confidence	5	4
Total	41	35

5 = highest, 1 = lowest.

interviews, and the new nurse's need to give several weeks notice of termination to the present employer, the hiring process should be initiated several months before the planned beginning of the nurse's employment and orientation (see Figure 4.2). If not already completed, new nurses will also need to take the 5-week Guided Care nursing course and obtain the Certificate in Guided Care Nursing before beginning work.

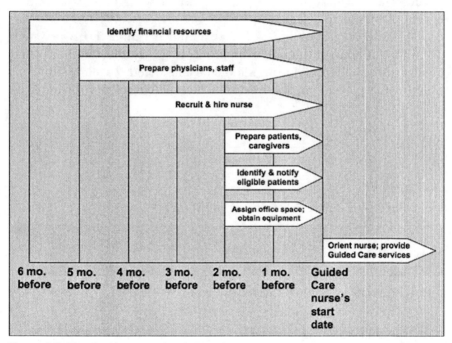

Figure 4.2 Timeline for launching Guided Care.

RESOURCE 4A: LETTER TO PATIENTS DESCRIBING GUIDED CARE

[Practice's letterhead]

[Date]

[Patient's full name]
[Address]
[City, State ZIP]

Dear [Mr./Ms. Last name]:

We are pleased to announce that we will soon offer a new service to our patients who have several chronic conditions. This new service, which is called Guided Care, will begin on [date].

What is Guided Care? In Guided Care, an experienced registered nurse works closely with you and your physician to assess your needs, plan how to meet those needs, monitor you and your health-related conditions, coordinate all the care you receive, help you care for yourself, support your family caregiver (if you have one), and connect you with services in the community that could help meet your needs.

Am I eligible to receive Guided Care? If insurance claims for health care you have received during the past year show that you have several chronic conditions that may require complex health care in the future, you will be eligible to receive Guided Care. If you are eligible, our Guided Care nurse will call you within a few months of [date] to offer to begin working with you and your physician to provide you these Guided Care services.

If I were eligible, would I be required to receive Guided Care? No, when the Guided Care nurse calls, you may say that you choose not to receive Guided Care. Choosing not to receive Guided Care would not affect your relationships with your physician, our practice or your insurer. Everything would continue as it is now.

If I were interested in Guided Care, what would happen next? You would select a convenient time for the Guided Care nurse to come to your home to talk with you and assess your health. During that visit, the nurse would explain the details of how Guided Care works. After you receive answers to all your questions, you would have time to talk with your family and friends before deciding whether to accept Guided Care. As before, choosing not to receive Guided Care would not affect your relationships with your physician, our practice or your insurer.

If I chose to receive Guided Care, what would happen next? The Guided Care nurse would work with your physician and you to create a plan for keeping you as healthy and independent as possible. From that time on, the nurse would offer you all the services listed in this letter. You would be free to accept or decline any of these services.

Would I have to pay extra to receive Guided Care services? No, there is no extra charge for Guided Care services. You would continue to be responsible, however, for the costs of any health care and other services you use that are not covered by your insurance.

We are offering Guided Care services to our patients who have several chronic conditions because we believe that these services will improve the quality of their health care and the quality of their lives. Our physicians, Guided Care nurse and other staff members are excited about working together to provide Guided Care. If our Guided Care nurse calls to offer you the option of receiving Guided Care, we hope you will give serious consideration to this opportunity.

[Signature]

[Name of medical director or practice administrator]

RESOURCE 4B: GUIDED CARE WAITING ROOM POSTER

> 66 My Guided Care nurse observed my conditions over time, even in my home, and gave me advice that I could not get from just an occasional visit to a doctor's office. 99
> Ben, Age 81

It's Like Having a Nurse in the Family

Lots of us have trouble managing our health conditions. With so many doctors, appointments, medicines and symptoms, a nurse in the family would help.

A Guided Care nurse will soon be part of this practice. The nurse will help some of our patients manage their medicines, doctor visits, insurance, and all health conditions. You may qualify for free support from our Guided Care nurse if you are over 65, have several chronic medical conditions, and agree to work with the Guided Care nurse.

If you are eligible, we will contact you soon with more information!

GUIDED CARE

CREDIT: Photo by Larry Canner.

RESOURCE 4C: JOB DESCRIPTION FOR GUIDED CARE NURSE

POSITION PROFILE/VACANCY ANNOUNCEMENT

POSITION TITLE: Guided Care nurse

Purpose:
To manage all aspects of patient-centered Guided Care for 50 to 60 frail elderly patients, working with one health care team. The nurse directly interfaces with physicians, health care teams, patients and their unpaid caregivers in managing patient care.

Accountabilities:
The ideal candidate will possess excellent interpersonal skills, with a flexible and creative approach to problems solving. The candidate will have a demonstrated ability of working effectively as a member of an interdisciplinary team, displaying good clinical judgment and decision-making skills. As a team member, the Guided Care nurse must possess excellent communication skills, both written and verbal, and an ability to listen and be assertive, as required. Central to the role of the Guided Care nurse is a commitment to "coaching" (rather than "teaching") patients to improve their health behaviors to attain their health-related goals. An ability to work independently is essential.

The Guided Care nurse will have a clear understanding of the role, and will demonstrate a commitment to implementation of the following accountabilities:

1. Comprehensive case management and care coordination for 50 to 60 frail elderly patients according to Guided Care principles. The Guided Care nurse is expected to provide the following services to each patient:
   a. Comprehensive geriatric home assessment
   b. Development and communication (with patient, caregiver and primary care physician/health care team) of a comprehensive care plan based on evidence-based best practice for chronic illness
   c. Pro-active management and follow-up (home visits and by telephone) according to care plan
   d. Management and coordination of all transitions in care:
      i. Communicate care plan to all providers in all settings of care (ED, hospital, rehabilitation facility, nursing home, home care and specialist)
      ii. Ensure that relevant providers receive timely clinical data for care treatment decisions in all settings of care (ED, hospital, rehabilitation facility, nursing home, home care and specialty care).
   e. Direct caregiver support, including ad hoc telephone advice
   f. Facilitation of patient and caregiver access to community resources relevant to patient's needs, including referrals to transportation programs, Meals on Wheels, senior centers, chore services, et cetera.
   g. Incorporation of self-care and shared decision making in all aspects of patient care.

Minimum requirements:
- Current licensure as a registered nurse in the state where the practice is located, and where the practice's patients live.
- Completion of an accredited course in Guided Care nursing (www.ijhn.jhmi.edu/calendar.asp). Tuition is free for nurses employed by practices participating in the Medicare Medical Home Demonstration.
- A Certificate in Guided Care Nursing issued by the American Nurses Credentialing Center.
- Three years of nursing experience, preferably with older patients.
- Proficient in computer use, the Internet, and health information technology.
- Ability to travel frequently to hospitals, skilled nursing facilities, patients' homes, and other sites where patients receive care (as indicated by patients' needs).

RESOURCE 4D: SAMPLE ADVERTISEMENT FOR GUIDED CARE NURSE

Recruiting registered nurses ◆ GUIDED **CARE**
for Guided Care ambulatory practice positions

Based at [Name of organization/primary care practice] in [Location], registered nurses will work with primary care physicians to provide the following ongoing services for 50 to 60 chronically ill older patients and their caregivers:

- Conduct comprehensive assessments in patients' homes
- Plan comprehensive chronic care collaboratively with physicians, patients and caregivers
- Monitor chronic conditions and coach patients and caregivers in self-management and lifestyle improvement
- Coordinate care among multiple providers
- Coordinate transitions between sites of care
- Facilitate access to community services
- Use health information technology

Applicant must be a licensed registered nurse with at least three years of nursing experience with older patients. He/she must have the ability to travel frequently to hospitals, skilled nursing facilities and patients' homes, and must be skilled in using computers, the Internet and health information technology.

To apply, please send cover letter and resume to [Name and address] or fax information to [000-000-000].

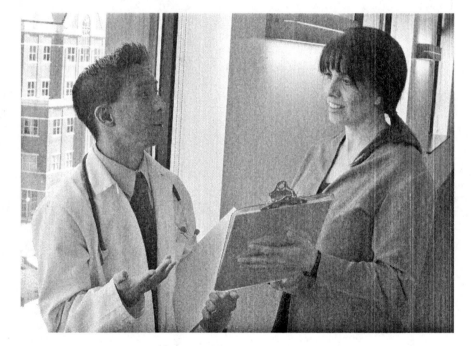

Photo 5.1 Guided Care nurse and a primary care physician discussing a new problem reported by a Guided Care patient.

CREDIT: Photo by Larry Canner.

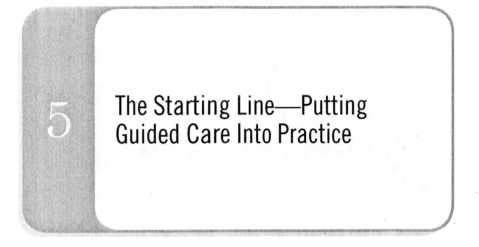

The Starting Line—Putting Guided Care Into Practice

After months of successful planning and preparation, the big day has finally arrived: It is the Guided Care nurse's first day of work in the practice. Like all new beginnings, it is a day of optimism and high hopes, and also one of some uncertainty and anxiety. A brief welcoming introduction of the nurse to the staff of the practice by the medical director and/or the practice administrator signals the practice's commitment to succeed with Guided Care. Each member of the staff should have already received a brief description of the goals of Guided Care, the role of the Guided Care nurse, and certain limitations to the nurse's scope of activities.

The *goals* of Guided Care are to maximize the quality of life for chronically ill patients and to maximize the quality and efficiency of their health care.

The *role* of the Guided Care nurse is to work in partnership with the primary care physician, the patient, the patient's caregiver, members of the office staff, and all other involved health care providers to attain the goals of Guided Care. This role includes eight primary activities, which are described in greater detail in chapter 2.

1. Assessing the patient at home.
2. Developing evidence-based plans for managing the patient's conditions and summarizing them in a Care Guide and an Action Plan.

3. Monitoring the patient's conditions and health-related behaviors monthly.
4. Engaging the patient in self-management.
5. Coordinating the efforts of all the professionals who provide health care to the patient.
6. Smoothing the patient's transitions between sites of health care, especially in and out of hospitals, skilled nursing facilities, and rehabilitation facilities.
7. Supporting the patient's caregiver, who may be a relative or a friend.
8. Facilitating access to supportive services in the community.

There are *limits* to the Guided Care nurse's role. Because of the time and effort required to provide these services to a caseload of 50 to 60 chronically ill patients, the Guided Care nurse is not able to fulfill other roles sometimes fulfilled by nurses. For example, the Guided Care nurse is not able to assist in the care of patients who do not qualify for Guided Care. For patients who do qualify, the Guided Care nurse performs only the above listed Guided Care services and does not even perform all of these services if another health care professional is available to provide them. For example, if a patient needed a referral to a community agency and a social worker were available, the nurse would ask the social worker to make the necessary arrangements. Or, if a patient needed home health care, the Guided Care nurse would facilitate a referral to a home health care agency and coordinate with the home care nurse(s), but would not provide the needed home care personally.

GUIDED CARE ORIENTATION

The next several months will be focused on orienting everyone in the practice, establishing a detailed individual plan for each Guided Care patient, and beginning to provide each patient with the full range of Guided Care services.

The first few weeks are devoted to building teamwork by orienting the nurse to the people and the procedures of the practice and by orienting the physicians and other staff members to the nurse and to the operational details of how Guided Care will work in the practice. The nurse's supervisor is responsible for planning and conducting this orientation. Depending on the size of the practice, this may be the practice administrator, the medical director, or another physician.

Components for the practice's Guided Care orientation are shown in Table 5.1, the Guided Care orientation checklist. Together, the supervisor and nurse plan the schedule and logistical arrangements for addressing all topics on the checklist. They meet weekly to review the nurse's progress and to make any necessary modifications. This orientation is complete when the nurse and the supervisor agree that all of the orientation topics have been addressed successfully.

Table 5.1

GUIDED CARE ORIENTATION CHECKLIST		
DATE COMPLETED	**SUPERVISOR'S/ NURSE'S INITIALS**	**ORIENTATION TOPIC**
		Developing effective teamwork with physicians
		First one-on-one orientation meeting with each physician
		Nurse observation of each physician's interactions with Guided Care patients during office visits
		Each physician's observation of the nurse's interactions with Guided Care patients
		Second one-on-one orientation meeting with each physician
		Establishing plans for periodic one-on-one physician meetings to improve teamwork
		Developing effective teamwork with members of the office staff
		The nurse acquires an understanding of:
		The roles of each member of the office staff
		The administrative relationships among all practice personnel
		The practice's processes for:
		Refilling prescriptions

(Continued)

Table 5.1

DATE COMPLETED	SUPERVISOR'S/ NURSE'S INITIALS	ORIENTATION TOPIC
		Arranging referrals
		Scheduling patients' appointments
		Reminding patients of appointments
		Notifying patients of test results
		Maintaining medical records (paper and electronic)
		Patient flow through the office
		Handling telephone messages
		Communicating with specific local hospitals and emergency departments about patients' admissions, discharges, and test results
		Contacting specific local health care professionals who often serve Guided Care patients: consultants, social workers, dieticians, pharmacists, health educators, rehab and skilled nursing facilities, home care agencies, and hospice
		Providing after-hours on-call services
		Collecting co-payments from patients
		Submitting claims to insurance companies
		Staff meetings and social events
		Personnel policies: paychecks, employee benefits, vacations, sick time, reimbursement for expenses, parking, identification badges, security of the office building

GUIDED CARE ORIENTATION CHECKLIST *(Continued)*

(Continued)

Table 5.1

GUIDED CARE ORIENTATION CHECKLIST *(Continued)*		
DATE COMPLETED	**SUPERVISOR'S/ NURSE'S INITIALS**	**ORIENTATION TOPIC**
		Completing necessary training in
		The use of the health information techonology that supports Guided Care
		Health Information and Patient Accountability Act (HIPAA)
		Performance of relevant clinical functions within the practice, for example, schoduling appointments, refilling prescriptions, and making referrals
		Creating an information database of community resources that serve Guided Care patients and caregivers
		The Area Agency on Aging, Meals on Wheels, senior centers, transportation programs, chore services, adult day health care centers, Alzheimer's Association, support groups, exercise programs, chronic disease self-management programs

As detailed in Table 5.1, the goals of the orientation are for the Guided Care nurse to begin to develop effective teamwork with the physician(s) and the other members of the office staff, as well as to become familiar with office procedures and health-related resources in the local community.

Building Teamwork With the Practice's Physician(s)

To begin building the essential nurse–physician teamwork, the nurse's supervisor schedules the first in a continuing series of one-on-one meetings between the nurse and individual physicians. In this meeting, the nurse and the physician define and discuss the many processes they will soon conduct as a team: refining each new patient's Preliminary Care Guide, sharing new knowledge about changes in outpatients' clinical status, informing each other about their mutual patients' transitions into and out of hospitals and other facilities, responding to calls from patients and their caregivers, coverage during vacations and other absences, and communicating with each other efficiently, for example, by e-mail, voice mail, in-person meetings, and entries in the medical record (see Table 5.2).

Initially, the nurse should shadow the physicians through their routine office encounters with newly identified Guided Care patients to be

Table 5.2

NURSE–PHYSICIAN TEAMWORK ACTIVITIES	
Updating each other about the status of patients	The Guided Care nurse provides the physician with a current list of their mutual Guided Care patients.
	The Guided Care nurse notifies the physician of significant changes in their mutual patients' status, especially changes occurring between office visits and during care in hospitals and skilled nursing facilities.
	The physician notifies the nurse of changes in their mutual patients' status, especially admissions to hospitals, visits to emergency departments, and referrals to specialists.
	Depending on personal preferences, notifications could occur by e-mail, voice mail, hard copy notes, direct conversations and/or entries in the medical record.
Providing care collaboratively	The Guided Care nurse and physician discuss and modify Preliminary Care Guides of patients who enroll in Guided Care.
	The nurse joins the physician in the examining room during office visits, especially with patients who have acute problems or difficulty with communication, cognition, and/or adherence, or who have recently received care in hospitals or emergency departments.
Quality improvement processes	The Guided Care nurse and the physician discuss ways to improve their Guided Care teamwork, and the nurse attends appropriate office staff meetings.

introduced to the patients as the physician's partner and to observe the physicians' styles of interacting with their patients. After the nurse has begun building a caseload, each physician should observe the nurse interacting with a sample of their mutual patients.

Over time, each nurse–physician team will develop its own unique style of teamwork. Refining effective teamwork is, however, a long, dynamic process that requires commitment, respect, flexibility, feedback, persistence, and patience by each party. Thus, even after Guided Care has been launched, the nurse and physician(s) should meet briefly, and regularly, to assess and improve the effectiveness of their teamwork.

Building Teamwork With the Practice's Office Staff

To build teamwork as a new member of the office staff, the Guided Care nurse must learn the roles of all the existing members of the office staff and the administrative relationships among them. The nurse meets with each staff member individually to explain the goals, role, and limits of the Guided Care nurse, as listed below, and to learn the roles of other members of the staff and how they conduct many important processes, including all those on the Guided Care orientation checklist. In doing so, the nurse builds a database of frequently used clinical resources in the community: hospitals, emergency departments, consultants, social workers, dieticians, pharmacists, health educators, rehabilitation and skilled nursing facilities, home care agencies, and hospice programs.

The agenda for these individual meetings includes: a description of the role of the staff member, a description of the duties of a Guided Care nurse, and a discussion of how the nurse will complement the role of the staff member. When the Guided Care nurse's tasks could potentially overlap with tasks performed by the other staff member (e.g., an office nurse or clerical person, or a practice-based social worker or pharmacist), the role of the Guided Care nurse is to communicate and coordinate with the other staff member, but not to assume any of the other person's responsibilities. A rule of thumb for Guided Care nurses' interactions with other health care workers is: "Collaborate with everyone, and displace no one." The Guided Care nurse also attends the regular meetings of the practice staff.

In addition to maintaining strong collaborative relationships with the physicians and staff members of the practice, the Guided Care nurse also needs ongoing professional interactions with other registered nurses, nurse care managers, and Guided Care nurses. Such interactions are available through the activities of local, state, and/or national profes-sional societies, such as the National Gerontological Nurses Association (NGNA), the Case Management Society of American (CMSA), and the American Nurses Association (ANA).

Training and Orientation to Community Resources

To complete the orientation, the nurse also obtains any training that is re-quired for clinical members of the staff, such as training and certification in the use of office computer systems and in the regulations of the Health Information and Patient Accountability Act (HIPAA). Finally, by talking with staff members and the leaders of the local Area Agency on Aging and other community agencies that serve older adults, the nurse com-piles a database of contact information for making patient and caregiver referrals to health-related nonmedical resources in the local community.

ESTABLISHING A PLAN FOR EACH GUIDED CARE PATIENT

While the practice is developing its Guided Care teamwork, the Guided Care nurse also begins to establish an individual comprehensive plan for each of 50 to 60 chronically ill patients of the practice who are eligible to receive Guided Care. The practice administrator gives the Guided Care nurse and the appropriate physician the names and contact information of all the practice's patients who have been classified as eligible to receive Guided Care. The process of establishing a comprehensive plan involves a 9-step sequence that usually requires 3 to 4 weeks to complete for each patient. While the team is building the caseload of Guided Care patients from 0 to 60, 5 to 10 patients are usually in the assessment process at all times, progressing through the following steps.

1. *Letter to patient.* The practice administrator mails a letter simi-lar to Resource 5A: Eligibility Letter to Patients at the end of the chapter to one or two eligible patients each week (with a copy sent to the nurse), notifying them that they are eligible (but not required) to receive Guided Care and that the practice's Guided Care nurse will call them within the next week.
2. *Call to patient.* The Guided Care nurse calls one or two eligible patients per week to provide more details about Guided Care, to answer their questions, to ask whether they are interested in

receiving Guided Care and, if appropriate, to schedule a time to visit their homes to assess their health status (see Resource 5B: Script of Guided Care Nurse's First Telephone Conversation With Patient). For patients who are interested, the nurse uses pages 1–2 of the Health History Form (Resource 5C) to perform a focused brief review of the patient's medical record at the practice. As indicated by Xs on page 1 of the history form, the patient's chronic conditions determine what physical findings and laboratory results the nurse seeks and records on condition-specific assessment forms (see Appendix B: Condition-Specific Assessment Forms).

3. *Consent.* The Guided Care nurse visits each interested patient's home to meet the patient, describe Guided Care, answer the patient's questions, invite the patient to accept Guided Care and, If appropriate, obtain the patient's signature on a consent and authorization for the release of medical information form (Resource 5D: Patient Consent and Authorization for the Release of Medical Information, located at the end of this chapter).

4. *Initial assessment of the patient.* After the patient signs the consent form, the nurse proceeds in conducting a comprehensive in-home assessment of the patient. For about 2 hours, the nurse follows pages 3–10 of the Health History Form (Resource 5C) in completing an in-depth interview with the patient and an evaluation of the safety and functionality of the patient's home environment.

5. *Initial assessment of the caregiver.* If, in the health history, the patient reports having a disability and identifies a family caregiver (or friend), the Guided Care nurse invites the caregiver by telephone to participate in the Guided Care education and support program for caregivers. If the caregiver accepts, the nurse sends the caregiver a confirming letter with an attached information form (similar to Resource 5E: Caregiver Invitation Letter and Resource 5F: Caregiver Assessment Form, respectively) that the caregiver completes independently. The nurse then discusses the information on the form with the caregiver during a structured 30-minute assessment at a prearranged time and place, often the patient's home but sometimes by telephone, if the caregiver requests). Sometimes these caregiver assessments can be completed immediately after the nurse's initial home assessment of the patient, if the caregiver is present and available.

6. *Preliminary Care Guide.* The nurse enters the patient assessment data collected from the home visit and from the patient's medical record into the practice's health information technology system and then generates a personalized, evidence-based, comprehensive Preliminary Care Guide (see Resource 2A, located at the end of chapter 2).

7. *Care Guide.* The nurse and the patient's primary care physician meet for 20 to 25 minutes to review and modify the Preliminary Care Guide to create a Care Guide that reflects not only the applicable evidence-based guidelines for managing the patient's chronic conditions, but also the patient's life expectancy, comorbidity, and stated preferences for health care and health-related behaviors (Resource 2B).

8. *Revision of the Care Guide.* The nurse discusses the Care Guide with the patient and caregiver and then revises it to make it consistent with the patient's intentions and capabilities—and to ensure that the patient and caregiver regard it as *their* plan. The nurse places the Care Guide in the medical record and uses it to communicate the plan for managing the patient's chronic conditions to each health care professional who treats the patient.

9. *Creation of the patient's Action Plan.* The nurse converts the Care Guide into a patient-friendly Action Plan, which expresses each desired action, such as taking medications and observing dietary restrictions, in the patient's language and in large print (see Resource 2C). The patient or caregiver displays the Action Plan prominently in a plastic jacket on the patient's refrigerator or cupboard, where it serves as a list of reminders of behaviors that will maximize the patient's health. The nurse also places an identification card (similar to Resource 5G: Guided Care Identification Card, located at the end of this chapter) with the Medicare or other health insurance card in the patient's wallet to alert health care providers to the availability of the nurse to provide them with the patient's clinical information and to help coordinate their care with that of other providers.

As the planning for each patient is completed, the practice team begins providing that patient and caregiver with all six services of ongoing Guided Care: monthly monitoring, coaching for self-management, coordinating care, smoothing transitions, supporting caregivers, and accessing community resources. As the planning is completed for more and more patients, more of the nurse's time is required to provide these patients with ongoing services, and less time is available for creating new plans for other patients. Thus, completing the planning phase expeditiously allows the team to focus on providing ongoing Guided Care to the entire caseload. Completing all 9 steps for a full panel of 50 to 60 Guided Care patients usually requires 6 to 8 months.

PROVIDING ONGOING GUIDED CARE EFFECTIVELY AND EFFICIENTLY

Even after the initial planning phase has been completed, providing comprehensive ongoing Guided Care effectively and efficiently to 50 to 60 patients, each of whom has several chronic conditions, can be challenging, especially during periods when several of these patients experience exacerbations of their chronic conditions and/or admission to hospitals simultaneously.

Four strategies allow the team to manage these episodes of intense demand for ongoing Guided Care services.

1. *Develop a reliable detection system* for the team to learn promptly whenever a Guided Care patient is admitted to a hospital. This allows the team to begin providing transitional care proactively. To overcome the poor communication inherent in today's fragmented health care, such a system must be multifaceted.

   - Patients and caregivers are urged to notify their Guided Care nurse whenever they go to a hospital or emergency department.
   - The Guided Care identification card (Resource 5G) in the patient's wallet requests hospital clerical personnel to call the nurse at the time of admission.
   - The admissions departments of local hospitals are given the names of all Guided Care patients so they can detect admissions electronically and send a fax or e-mail notice to the team within hours.
   - The practice's physicians and office staff members are asked to inform the Guided Care nurse immediately whenever a Guided Care patient has been admitted to a hospital.

2. *Set limits* on the services provided. Among the many useful services the nurse could provide for Guided Care patients, the six services that constitute ongoing Guided Care (the services that follow the initial assessment and the creation of a Care Guide

and Action Plan) have the highest priority. Even when providing these services, the nurse must limit the amount of time devoted to each patient and each service. For example, longitudinal psychological counseling of patients or caregivers by the nurse is rarely possible. The practice's physicians and other staff members can help the nurse to observe these limits by reinforcing them during their meetings together.

3. *Share responsibility* with other appropriate resources. For example, the nurse might suggest that a capable caregiver call the local Area Agency on Aging for guidance in selecting an adult day health care center, rather than providing such guidance personally.

4. *Prioritize demands* for Guided Care services. On days when the nurse cannot provide all routine ongoing services to all Guided Care patients, the nurse gives top priority to providing two services that are most crucial to the immediate well-being of the patient: providing transitional care, and attending to exacerbations of chronic conditions and the emergence of acute problems.

RESOURCE 5A: ELIGIBILITY LETTER TO PATIENTS

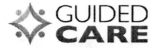

[Date]

Dear [Mr./Mrs./Ms. last name],

You have the opportunity to participate in a program [Name of practice] is offering. The program, called Guided Care, provides patients with a nurse who gives them information about their health problems, helps them obtain health-related services, and coordinates all their health care. You are eligible for this program because you have chronic conditions that may require medical care in the future.

As a participant in this program, you will continue to receive regular care from me, plus you will get a Guided Care Nurse. This nurse will work closely with you and me to provide you with extra services. It is important to understand that the Guided Care nurse will not substitute or take the place of me, or any of your other doctors or care providers.

Participating in this program is your choice. Within the next two weeks, [Name of nurse], our Guided Care nurse, will call you and ask to come to your home to do an analysis of your health. When she is in your home, she will ask for your permission to be in this program and she will ask you questions about your health and history of health care. When that is completed, she will work closely with me, to develop a care plan that is specific to you and your health conditions. She will be in touch with you at least monthly to check on you, and she will help coordinate your care if you see other doctors or go to the hospital. If you do not want to take part in this program, please call [000-000-000], and we will remove you from our list.

Thank you for considering this program.

[Primary care physician's name, signature]

RESOURCE 5B: SCRIPT OF GUIDED CARE NURSE'S FIRST TELEPHONE CONVERSATION WITH PATIENT

Introduction

Hello, I am [name]. I am a registered nurse calling from [physician's name]'s office. Recently you should have received a letter from our office telling you that you are eligible to receive a new service we are offering at no cost to you. It's called Guided Care, and I am calling now to talk to you about what Guided Care is and to answer your questions about it.

Background

Guided Care is health care from your doctor, plus extra help from me. Your doctor and I work together as a team. Between your regular visits with your doctor, I will do several things for you:

- I will be available by cell phone Monday through Friday from 9 a.m. to 5 p.m. to answer your questions, check with your doctor, give you advice, and help you get the health-related services you need.
- I will help you to make a practical plan for staying as healthy and independent as possible, and I will help you to follow your plan.
- I will coordinate all the health care you receive from hospitals, doctors, and other health care professionals.
- I will help any of your family or friends who help you.
- If you go into a hospital, I will visit you in the hospital, and I will visit you soon after you go home just to make sure everything is going smoothly.
- I will help you to take advantage of other special services in your neighborhood, such as help with transportation, meals, home modifications, and physical activity.

Do you have any questions about Guided Care?

Choice

Of course, you are not required to accept these extra Guided Care services. You could choose to continue receiving health care from your doctor as before without any help from me. Would you like to learn more about how you can receive Guided Care?

If "no" – Thanks for considering it. Please tell your doctor if you would like to reconsider.

If "yes," proceed with enrollment.

Enrollment

To get started, I would like to meet with you and any of your family and friends who help you. I could come out to your home or, if you would prefer, we could meet the first time at Dr. [Last name]'s office. Some time soon, I would like to spend about two hours getting to know all about you and your health. Is there a time that would be convenient for me to visit you at home?

RESOURCE 5C: HEALTH HISTORY FORM

> Place Patient
> ID # Here

Medical Record (Completed before home visit for Initial Assessments)

DOB_____ Age_____ Identifier_____ e-mail address _____
Address_____ Phone_____

(T) Conditions

Congestive Heart Failure (CHF)	Dementia	Falling	Osteoporosis (OP)
Constipation	Depression	Hypertension (HTN)	Persistent pain
COPD/asthma	Diabetes (DM)	Insomnia	Urinary incontinence
Coronary artery disease (CAD)	Disability	Osteoarthritis (OA)	Other:

	Most Recent Date	Value	CHF	COPD	CAD	Dem	DM	HTN	OA	OP	Pain	H.M
Height	_/_/_	ft__in										M/F
Weight	_/_/_	lbs										M/F
BP	_/_/_		X	X	X			X				
Heart Rate (pulse)	_/_/_		X	X	X							
Crackles	_/_/_		X									
Pedal Edema	_/_/_		X									
BUN	_/_/_		X				X	X	X			
Creatinine	_/_/_		X				X	X	X			
Potassium (K)	_/_/_		X					X				
ALT	_/_/_										X	
AST	_/_/_										X	
Total cholesterol	_/_/_						X	X				M/F
LDL	_/_/_						X	X				M/F
HDL	_/_/_						X	X				M/F
Triglycerides	_/_/_						X	X				M/F
HgA1c	_/_/_						X					
TSH	_/_/_						X					F
B12	_/_/_					X						
Oxygen saturation	_/_/_		X					X				
Creatinine clearance	_/_/_		X				X	X				
Urinary protein	_/_/_											
FEV1	_/_/_			X								
X-ray—chest	_/_/_		X	X								
X-ray—joint/bone	_/_/_									X		
CT/MRI of head	_/_/_					X						
Mammogram	_/_/_											F
EKG	_/_/_		X		X							
Ejection fraction	_/_/_		X		X							
Stress test	_/_/_				X							
Angiogram	_/_/_				X		X					
Dilated retinal exam	_/_/_						X					
Glucose (finger stick)	_/_/_											
Bone density	_/_/_									X		F
Colon/ sigmoidoscopy	_/_/_											M/F
Stool blood	_/_/_											M/F

(T) T-score < –1.5 triggers an initial assessment of osteoporosis

(Continued)

RESOURCE 5C: HEALTH HISTORY FORM *(Continued)*

	Place Patient ID # Here

Chronic Medications

Name	Dose	Route	Freq	Discrepancy	Nature	Reason	Notes

Overall adherence   GOOD   FAIR   POOR

Important allergies and other adverse reactions to medications

Substance: _____ Reaction: _____ Year: _____

Substance: _____ Reaction: _____ Year: _____

Substance: _____ Reaction: _____ Year: _____

Substance: _____ Reaction: _____ Year: _____

Medical History

Hospitalizations in past 2 years:

Hospital	Reason	Month/year
		/
		/
		/
		/

Pneumoccocal Vaccination: year_____

RESOURCE 5C: HEALTH HISTORY FORM *(Continued)*

Place Patient
ID # Here

In Home Assessment

Date visited ___/___/200__

Health problems of greatest importance to patient:
1. _____
2. _____
3. _____

/21 Nutrition (0-21)	/4 Cage (0-4)
/15 GDS (0-15)	/10 Pain (0-10)
/30 MMSE (0-30)	sec. Get Up & Go
P/F Screen for hearing loss	

Family and Friends

Name	Phone	Notes	CG	Emergency	DPOAHC	Doc on chart
_____	_____	_____				
_____	_____	_____				
_____	_____	_____				
_____	_____	_____				

Insurance coverage

	Policy No.	Effective Date	Telephone	Notes:
Medicare A	_____	___/___/___	_____	_____
Medicare B	_____	___/___/___	_____	_____
Medicare D	_____	___/___/___	_____	_____
Medigap:	_____	___/___/___	_____	_____
Medicaid:	_____	___/___/___	_____	_____
Other:	_____	___/___/___	_____	_____

Do you experience a financial strain related to using any of these health services?		
Hospital, home care	No	Yes
Physician services, tests	No	Yes
Prescription medications	No	Yes

(Continued)

RESOURCE 5C: HEALTH HISTORY FORM *(Continued)*

> Place Patient
> ID # Here

Care providers (recent)	Most recent visit	Discipline	Phone	E-mail
Dr. _____	_____ / _____	primary care	__ - __ - ____	_____
_____	_____ / _____	Guided Care nurse	__ - __ - ____	_____
_____	_____ / _____	_____	__ - __ - ____	_____
_____	_____ / _____	_____	__ - __ - ____	_____
_____	_____ / _____	_____	__ - __ - ____	_____

Service providers (active)	Provider	Frequency	Phone	Notes
meals	_____	_____	__ - __ - ____	
transportation	_____	_____	__ - __ - ____	
chores	_____	_____	__ - __ - ____	
day care	_____	_____	__ - __ - ____	
cleaning	_____	_____	__ - __ - ____	
other	_____	_____	__ - __ - ____	
none				

Daily life

Actual diet consumed

salt-restricted
low-fat
diabetic
high-fiber
weight-reduction
calcium-enriched
other: _____
unrestricted

Exercise:

walking/other aerobic: _____ ___ min ___ times/week
resistance: _____ ___ min ___ times/week
balance: _____ ___ min ___ times/week
other: _____ ___ min ___ times/week
none

Religion

Subscribe to a religion?   No   Yes: _____

If yes, importance in health matters?   low   medium   high

Tobacco & Alcohol Use

Tobacco present use:
   No
   Yes → ___ packs/day
Alcohol present use:
   No
   Yes → ___ drinks/week

Other

(T) Satisfied with sleep:
Yes   **No**   'No' triggers Initial Assessment of **Insomnia**.

(T) Urinary leakage restricts activity:
No   **Yes**   'Yes' triggers Initial Assessment of **Incontinence**.

(T) Falls in the past 6 months: #
'1' triggers Initial Assessment for **Falls**.

(T) Fractures in the past year:
No   Yes   'Yes' triggers Initial Assessment of **Osteoporosis**.

RESOURCE 5C: HEALTH HISTORY FORM *(Continued)*

<table>
<tr><td></td><td>Place Patient
ID # Here</td></tr>
</table>

Activities of Daily Living			
Do you usually *receive help or have difficulty* with:	YES	NO	N/A
Going places out of walking distance, including traveling on buses, taxis, or in a car?			
Shopping for groceries?			
Preparing your meals, including planning and cooking your meals?			
Doing housework or light cleaning, such as dusting or washing dishes?			
Bathing, or getting in and out of the tub or shower?			
Dressing, including choosing and putting on your clothes?			
Using the toilet, including getting to the bathroom, cleaning yourself, arranging your clothes, or managing a bedpan or commode?			
Getting in and out of bed or chairs?			
Eating, including cutting meat, buttering bread, or opening containers?			
Walking across a room?			
(T) 'Yes' answer to any question *above* triggers an Initial Assessment for **Disability**.			
Does anyone *usually help you* with:	Yes	No	N/A
Managing your health care, including getting medicines or visiting/talking with doctors?			
Taking your medication, including help with reminders, correct doses, correct times, or setting up pills?			
Using the telephone, including looking up numbers and dialing?			
Handling your money, including writing checks and paying bills?			

If any 'yes' responses (to the 14 questions above):
    Who helps you the most with these activities: a relative, an acquaintance, paid help?
    _____
 	
If a relative or an unpaid acquaintance:
    May I invite him/her to participate? No Yes → Name:_____ Phone #:_____			

(Continued)

RESOURCE 5C: HEALTH HISTORY FORM *(Continued)*

Tour of home

Lighting inadequate:			
daytime	Yes	No	
nighttime	Yes	No	
Hazards for tripping:			
surfaces	Yes	No	
cords		No	
objects	Yes	No	
other:			
Slippery surfaces:			
tub/shower	Yes	No	
other:	Yes	No	
Stairs in need of rails:	Yes	No	
Telephone: inaccessible	Yes	No	
Smoke detector(s):			
absent	Yes	No	
non-functional	Yes	No	

(T) Physical barrier(s) to entry?
   Yes 'Yes' triggers an Initial Assessment for **Disability**
   No

(T) Physical barrier(s) inside home?
   Yes 'Yes' triggers an Initial Assessment for **Disability**.
   No

(T) Stove safe?
   Yes
   N 'No' triggers an Initial Assessment for **Disability**.

Devices and Equipment

(T) If 'not functional', triggers suggestion for referral

Place Patient ID # Here

Reason (if not functional)

	Needed		Present		Functional		Defective	Mismatched	Technique	Other	Reasons
Glasses	Yes	No	Yes	No	Yes	No					_____
Hearing aid	Yes	No	Yes	No	Yes	No					_____
Brace	Yes	No	Yes	No	Yes	No					_____
Prosthesis	Yes	No	Yes	No	Yes	No					_____
Cane	Yes	No	Yes	No	Yes	No					_____
Walker	Yes	No	Yes	No	Yes	No					_____
Wheelchair	Yes	No	Yes	No	Yes	No					_____
Hospital bed	Yes	No	Yes	No	Yes	No					_____
Tub/shower			Yes	No	Yes	No					_____
Bath bench	Yes	No	Yes	No	Yes	No					_____
Hand shower	Yes	No	Yes	No	Yes	No					_____
Raised seat	Yes	No	Yes	No	Yes	No					_____
Grab bar(s)	Yes	No	Yes	No	Yes	No					_____
Commode	Yes	No	Yes	No	Yes	No					_____
Other:	Yes	No	Yes	No	Yes	No					_____

Impressions

_____

_____

_____

RESOURCE 5C: HEALTH HISTORY FORM *(Continued)*

	Place Patient ID # Here

Nutrition

I'm going to read 10 statements about meals. Please tell me if each statement is true or false:

	True/False	True
I have an illness or condition that made me change the kind and/or amount of food I eat.		2
I eat fewer than 2 meals a day.		3
I eat few fruits, vegetables, or milk products.		2
I have 3 or more drinks of beer, liquor, or wine almost every day.		2
I have tooth or mouth problems that make it hard for me to eat.		2
I don't always have enough money to buy the food I need.		4
I eat alone most of the time.		1
I take 3 or more different prescribed or over-the-counter drugs a day.		1
Without wanting to, I have lost or gained 10 pounds.		2
I am not always physically able to shop, cook, and feed myself.		2
	Total (0-21)	___

(T) A score of > 3 suggests a referral for evaluation by a dietician.

Mini Mental Status Exam (MMSE)

	Scale	Points
Orientation:		
What is the year, season, date, day, month?	0-5	
Where are we (country, state, county, city, building)?	0-5	
Registration:		
Repeat the names of three objects: apple, pencil, chair.	0-3	
Attention:		
Begin with 100 and count backwards by 7 (stop after 5 answers).	0-5	
Or, spell the word "world" backwards.		
Recall:		
Ask for the names of the three objects.	0-3	
Language:		
Show a pencil and a watch and ask patient to name them.	0-2	
Repeat this phrase: "No ifs, ands, or buts."	0-1	
Please take this paper in your right hand, fold it in half, and put it on the floor.	0-3	
Read and obey this sentence: (show the sentence, "CLOSE YOUR EYES").	0-1	
Write a sentence.	0-1	
Visual-spatial:		
Copy this drawing as accurately as you can: (show intersecting pentagons).	0-1	
Total (0-30)		___

(T) A score < 25 triggers an Initial Assessment of **Dementia**

(Continued)

RESOURCE 5C: HEALTH HISTORY FORM *(Continued)*

Place Patient
ID # Here

● ●

Pain

On a scale of 0-10, with 0 being no pain and 10 being the most intense pain possible, how would you rate the severity of pain you had on most days of the past month?

Score (0-10):____

(**T**) A score of 3+ triggers an Initial Assessment of **Persistent Pain**.

● ●

Feelings

	Yes/No	Key	Match (1 pt)
Are you basically satisfied with your life?		No	
Have you dropped many of your activities and interests?		Yes	
Do you feel that your life is empty?		Yes	
Do you often get bored?		Yes	
Are you in good spirits most of the time?		No	
Are you afraid that something bad is going to happen to you?		Yes	
Do you feel happy most of the time?		No	
Do you often feel helpless?		Yes	
Do you often prefer to stay home at night, rather than go out and do new things?		Yes	
Do you feel that you have more problems with memory than most?		Yes	
Do you think it is wonderful to be alive now?		No	
Do you feel pretty worthless the way you are now?		Yes	
Do you feel full of energy?		No	
Do you feel your situation is hopeless?		Yes	
Do you think that most persons are better off than you?		Yes	
	Total (0-15)		

Score one point for each response that matches the 'yes' or 'no' answer after the question.

(**T**) A score of 5+ triggers an Initial Assessment of **Depression**.

RESOURCE 5C: HEALTH HISTORY FORM *(Continued)*

	Place Patient ID # Here

CAGE   **Yes/No**

Have you ever felt you should <u>C</u>ut down on your drinking?	
Have people <u>A</u>nnoyed you by criticizing your drinking?	
Have you ever felt bad or <u>G</u>uilty about drinking?	
Have you ever taken a drink first thing in the morning (<u>E</u>ye opener) to steady your nerves or get rid of a hangover?	
Each Yes = 1 point Total (0-4)	_____

○○○

Screen for hearing loss

Can you usually hear and understand what a person says without seeing his/her face, if that person <u>talks to you in a normal voice</u> from across the room (using your hearing aid, if you have one)?
☐ Yes   ☐ No
Can you usually hear and understand what a person says without seeing his/her face, if that person whispers to you from across the room (using your hearing aid, if you have one)?
☐ Yes   ☐ No   If no, skip the next question.
(T) A "no" answer to either question suggests a referral for evaluation by an audiologist.

○○○

Instructions
Equipment needed: watch with second hand and a standard arm chair
Be sure the patient is using his/her usual footwear, walking aid, and any sensory aids (e.g., glasses, hearing aid).
Instruct patient
   This is a short test of your basic ability to move about. We will practice before we conduct the test. I would like you to sit with your back against the chair, place your arms on the chair's arms, place your walking aid (if any) in position to use. Now, on the word "Go", please:

Get up & Go
   Walk at a comfortable speed to the line (3 meters/10 feet).
   Turn around.
   Walk back to the chair.
   Sit down.

<u>Time:</u>	___ seconds		
<u>Balance:</u>	normal	abnormal	
<u>Effective use of ambulatory aid:</u>	yes	no	N/A

(T) A time of > 20 seconds **or** abnormal balance **or** ineffective use of aid triggers Initial Assessment for **Falls**.

(Continued)

RESOURCE 5C: HEALTH HISTORY FORM *(Continued)*

Place Patient
ID # Here

Referrals recommended:
- ☐ optometry
- ☐ audiology
- ☐ dietician
- ☐ PT
- ☐ OT
- ☐ orthotist

Guided Care nurse recommendations
- ☐ lighting: _____
- ☐ hazards for tripping: _____
- ☐ slippery surfaces: _____
- ☐ stair rails: _____
- ☐ telephone access: _____ ˙
- ☐ smoke detectors: _____

RESOURCE 5D: PATIENT CONSENT/AUTHORIZATION FOR THE RELEASE OF MEDICAL INFORMATION

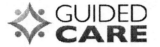

[Date]

I, [patient's name], am a participant in the Guided Care program. As a Guided Care participant, I understand that I will work closely with a Guided Care nurse, who will provide the following services:

1. The Guided Care nurse will come to my home to get information about my health, medical history, my ability to do usual activities and my social situation. From this information, the nurse and my primary care doctor will work with me to develop an individualized plan for treating each of my health problems. This plan will be put on a computer to guide all the doctors who take care of me.
2. The Guided Care nurse will provide education and coaching about following a healthy life style and using medication properly.
3. The Guided Care nurse will help coordinate the work of all the doctors and other health care professionals involved in my care.
4. The Guided Care nurse will help me to find and use community services that may be helpful to me.
5. The Guided Care nurse will call me or I will call him/her about once a month to see how I am doing and to recommend changes such as in diet, medication or activities if necessary. If I am having health problems, the nurse might call more often.

As part of the Guided Care Program, I hereby authorize release of my medical record information by health care providers who have treated me or reviewed or analyzed my health care data. The health care provider(s) will be identified during talks with my Guided Care nurse. The purpose or need for such disclosure is to accurately assess and provide continuity of my care. My Guided Care nurse is [name of nurse]. Requested reports and documents can be faxed to my Guided Care nurse at [nurse's fax number].

This authorization does not expire. The following documents may be released:

▨	Inpatient records	▨	EKG
▨	Emergency department records	▨	Cath report
▨	Outpatient records	▨	Cardiology studies
▨	Lab tests	▨	Discharge summaries
▨	Operative reports	▨	Mental health record
▨	Other:		

Signature: **Date:**

If anyone other than the patient signs this form, please complete the following:

I _____ represent that I am the health care agent/guardian of the patient.
       (Print name)   (Circle one of the above)

If you are the health care agent or guardian, please provide proof of your authority to act on behalf of the patient.

RESOURCE 5E: CAREGIVER INVITATION LETTER

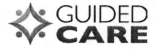

[Date]

Dear Mr./Mrs./Ms. [caregiver's name]:

Thank you for your interest in taking part in Guided Care. I am looking forward to meeting you and working with you to better care for your [Guided Care patient's relationship to caregiver].

The goal of Guided Care is to help the person for whom you provide care, as well as you, over time. For this reason, I have contacted you to schedule some time to meet with you. It would be helpful if you could complete the following information before we meet. *We ask that you have the attached form completed and with you at the time of our meeting.* Your responses will be used by me and your [Guided Care patient's relationship to caregiver]'s physician to better understand how to meet your needs.

Lastly, I wanted to confirm that we have agreed to meet at [Time] on [Date], at [Location]. Our meeting will take approximately 30 minutes. If you should have any questions or concerns before we meet, feel free to reach me at [contact number]. I look forward to meeting you in person!

Warm regards,

_____

Guided Care nurse

P.S. Please complete the attached form before our appointment.

RESOURCE 5F: CAREGIVER ASSESSMENT FORM

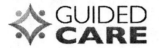

Information about you:

1. Name _____

2. Street address _____

3. City and ZIP _____

4. Home phone _____

5. Work phone _____
    (if applicable)

6. Other phone _____
    (if applicable)

7. E-mail address _____
    (if applicable)

8. Age _____

9. Gender   Male   ☐

               Female   ☐

10. Language spoken _____
    (if other than English)

11. Marital status _____

12. Employment   Full Time   ☐

                 Part Time   ☐

                 Neither   ☐

13. Number of children _____

14. Ages of children _____;   _____;   _____;

15. How do you usually travel about town?

    I drive.   ☐

    I am driven by others.   ☐

    I use public transportation.   ☐

(Continued)

RESOURCE 5F: CAREGIVER ASSESSMENT FORM *(Continued)*

16. In general, my health is:

      Excellent   ☐

      Very good   ☐

      Good   ☐

      Fair   ☐

      Poor   ☐

17. Were you seen by a medical provider in the last six months?

      Yes   ☐

      No   ☐

      If no, when was the last time you were seen by a medical provider?

      _____

18. We are interested in knowing if you have any health problems of your own. Please list any serious health conditions or physical difficulties in performing daily activities that you have.

      _____

      _____

19. How are you related to Mr./Mrs./Ms. [Guided Care patient's name]? I am their:

      Spouse/partner   ☐

      Son   ☐

      Daughter   ☐

      Son-in-law   ☐

      Daughter-in-law   ☐

      Brother   ☐

      Sister   ☐

      Grandchild   ☐

      Neighbor   ☐

      Other: _____

20. Length of time helping: _____ years, or _____ months

21. Average time spent helping per week: _____ hours (all the time = 168 hours)

22. Do you live together?
      Yes   ☐

      No   ☐

23. If you do not live together, how long does it usually take for you to get to their home?
                      _____minutes

RESOURCE 5F: CAREGIVER ASSESSMENT FORM *(Continued)*

24. Number of people living in your household: _____

What are their relationships to you?

_____

_____

_____

_____

25. Sometimes family and friends help older adults. Tell us what Mr./Mrs./Ms. [Guided Care patient's name] needs help with, and who, if anyone, helps them. Check as many as apply:

Activities:	No help needed	I help	Others help
Feeding			
Dressing			
Bathing/showering			
Helping with the toilet			
Getting around inside			
Preparing meals			
Shopping/errands			
Laundry			
Housecleaning			
Making phone calls			
Paying bills/balancing checkbook			
Help with medications (obtaining, administering, making dose-change decisions)			
Monitoring symptoms and health			
Managing medical finances, bills, & forms?			
Scheduling medical appointments			
Accompanying to medical appointments			
Arranging or providing transportation to appointments			
Talking with physicians and nurses			
Keeping Mr./Mrs./Ms. [Guided Care patient's name] safe?			

If others help, who?   _____

(name and relationship to Guided Care patient)

_____

(name and relationship to Guided Care patient)

_____

(name and relationship to Guided Care patient)

(Continued)

RESOURCE 5F: CAREGIVER ASSESSMENT FORM *(Continued)*

26. In the event that there is an emergency and you are not available, we would like to know how to get in touch with another person (family member or interested friend) who knows your [relationship to Guided Care patient]. Please list the name and phone number of at least one other family or friend and their relationship to Mr./Mrs./Ms. [Guided Care patient]:

_____

(name, relationship, and phone number)

_____

(name, relationship, and phone number)

_____

(name, relationship, and phone number)

_____

(name, relationship, and phone number)

27. How would you rate your level of stress related to helping?

None _____   Low _____   Medium _____   High _____

28. When under stress, some people might increase their use of alcohol and drugs – even prescription drugs. Is this a concern for you, or has someone you know expressed concern?

Yes   ☐

No   ☐

Please indicate which services you currently use and which you would be interested in using if they were available	No need for service	Currently using service	Not using, but could be interested if available
Personal or nursing care services			
Housework service			
Transportation service			
Help with home modifications (ramp/wider door)			
Home delivered meals			
Adult day care			
Counseling or peer support			
A central place to go/call to find out what help is available			
Caregiver education or conferences			
One-on-one training			
Respite care services ("time off" from providing assistance)			

RESOURCE 5F: CAREGIVER ASSESSMENT FORM *(Continued)*

We are also interested in your need for information and training. Please indicate whether any of the following would be helpful to you.

1. Financial and legal information

   Information about Medicare _____

   Information about Medicare Part D (RX) _____

   Information about Medicaid _____

   Information about advanced directives and living wills _____

2. Information about specific chronic conditions

   General information _____

   Managing symptoms _____

   How to monitor conditions _____

   What to expect _____

   Caring for someone with dementia _____

3. Training for specialized tasks that you assume

   Lifting techniques _____

   Correct operation of medical equipment _____

   Correct use of assistive devices (e.g., walker) _____

   Medication management _____

   Changing a diaper _____

   Inspecting skin _____

   Taking blood pressure, pulse, counting respirations _____

4. Help to better cope with the stresses of caregiving

   How to manage stress _____

   Learning to relax and balance my life _____

   Learning how to ask for help _____

   How to solve problems related to caregiving _____

Rewards and challenges:

What qualities and personal strengths do you bring to your role in helping your [relationship to Guided Care patient]?

_____

_____

_____

What have you found to be rewarding about your role in providing help?

_____

_____

_____

(Continued)

RESOURCE 5F: CAREGIVER ASSESSMENT FORM *(Continued)*

What are the problems or difficulties you experience in providing help?

_____

_____

_____

Thinking about any challenges you face. Please list the one issue you would most like to change or for which you could most use assistance.

_____

_____

_____

If a class for Guided Care families and friends was offered to you, what times would be the most convenient for you to attend?

Day(s) of week: _____

                         _____

Time(s) of day: _____

                         _____

Other comments: _____

RESOURCE 5G: GUIDED CARE IDENTIFICATION CARD

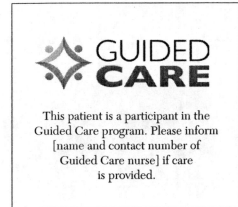

This patient is a participant in the
Guided Care program. Please inform
[name and contact number of
Guided Care nurse] if care
is provided.

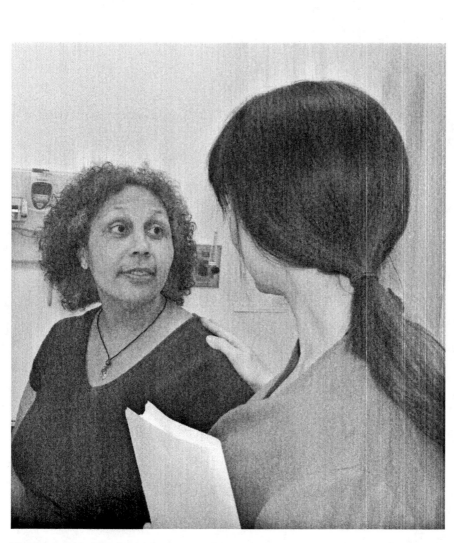

Photo 6.1 A Guided Care nurse conducting a motivational interview with a Guided Care patient.

CREDIT: Photo by Larry Canner.

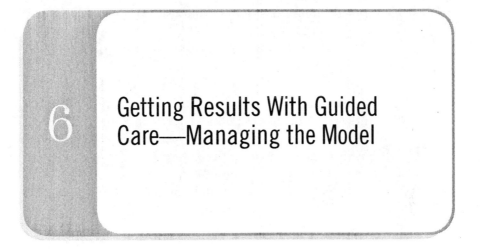

Getting Results With Guided Care—Managing the Model

Studies suggest that Guided Care works during the first 8 months of a randomized trial. In 14 community-based primary care teams, it improved the quality of patient care, and it reduced health care costs, largely a result of using less inpatient care. These savings more than offset the cost of the nurses. Guided Care also is popular with physicians, nurses, patients, and caregivers. A legitimate question, however, is, "How can we ensure that Guided Care will work in *our* practice?" How can we incorporate Guided Care into the unique circumstances of our environment, so that we get outcomes that are similar to those reported in research studies?

Success in translating Guided Care from the research setting to the real world depends on each practice's ability to conduct four interrelated processes:

1. A skilled leader within the practice—perhaps the practice administrator or medical director—must be identified as a committed "champion" for change. This person should be respected by the practice's personnel and committed to implementing Guided Care.

2. An accurate assessment must be made of the practice's readiness to adopt Guided Care. As described in chapter 3, the leader(s)

of the practice must determine whether the practice has (or can acquire) the necessary number of eligible patients, office space, health information technology, supporting revenue, and organizational commitment.

3. Careful preparation of all involved parties and components— patients, caregivers, physicians, office staff, and practice infrastructure—must be made before launching Guided Care. As emphasized in chapter 4, selecting a Guided Care nurse who is well-qualified and compatible with the practice's physicians and staff members is especially important.

4. The practice's champion for change must lead the practice assessment, the preparation, and the launching of Guided Care, and then use sound management principles to supervise the nurse and coordinate the Guided Care services provided by the practice.

This chapter briefly describes these essential management processes, and it offers suggestions for conducting them successfully. The first management process is to identify and acknowledge a leader within the practice as the local champion for the Guided Care transformation. Depending on the practice's size, ownership, resources, and geographic location, the champion may be a practice administrator, a medical director, another physician, or another member of the practice personnel. Regardless of who is selected for this role, the champion must have the requisite knowledge, skills, enthusiasm, commitment, experience, responsibility, credibility, authority, and accountability to develop Guided Care successfully within the practice.

As described earlier, the champion leads the practice through the processes of assessing its readiness for Guided Care (chapter 3), preparing to adopt Guided Care (chapter 4), and launching Guided Care (chapter 5).

At the core of these responsibilities is hiring and orienting the Guided Care nurse and integrating the Guided Care model into the operation of the practice. As the immediate supervisor, the champion facilitates the nurse's entry into the practice, providing a clear description of the nurse's responsibilities within the practice and the level of performance expected by the practice. The supervisor tracks data regularly that reflect the nurse's performance and communicates these data periodically as performance feedback to the nurse to reinforce desired behavior. The supervisor is also the person most responsible for communicating information about

Guided Care with insurers and with the practice's physicians, patients, and staff.

At first, the Guided Care nurse's role is new to everyone, so the supervisor must communicate a clear, consistent description of this role to all involved parties: patients, caregivers, physicians, office staff, and, most importantly, the nurse. This process of defining the nurse's role begins when the position is advertised and applicants are interviewed. Because the position is novel and multifaceted, providing a brief written description of the primary duties included in the job helps applicants to obtain a clear understanding of the position (Boyd et al., 2007).

Throughout the newly hired nurse's orientation, which the supervisor coordinates, the nurse clarifies the operational details of Guided Care during conversations with the primary care physicians, the office staff, the patients, and their caregivers. In these conversations, the nurse explains the eight primary activities within the Guided Care nurse's role, and the practice personnel explain how the practice operates. Together they integrate Guided Care into the practice.

Also during the orientation, the supervisor gives the nurse a clear set of expectations for ongoing performance in three domains:

■ *Building the initial caseload* of Guided Care patients: The nurse should begin this 9-step process (described in chapter 5) for about two patients each week and complete the process for about two other patients each week until the full caseload of 50 to 60 patients has been established. Progress through these steps will be slow at first, but it will accelerate as the nurse and the primary care physicians become increasingly familiar with the process.

■ *Developing teamwork* with each primary care physician in the practice: Building on the nurse's discussions with physicians about teamwork during orientation, the nurse should continue to meet briefly monthly or bimonthly with each physician to assess and improve the effectiveness of their teamwork. These meetings are distinct from discussions about specific patients. As Guided Care patients encounter other health care providers, such as specialty physicians, emergency department staff, and home care nurses, the Guided Care nurse also explains to them how Guided Care can complement their efforts. Providing these health care professionals with a brief verbal and written description of the relevant components of the Guided Care nurse's role (see Table 6.1) reinforces this message.

Table 6.1

HOW DOES A GUIDED CARE NURSE HELP?

Definition of Guided Care nurse	A registered nurse who specializes in working with physicians and other health care professionals to optimize the care of patients with chronic conditions.
Guided Care nurse's roles	Provides all health professionals with current comprehensive summaries of their patients' health status and management plans.
	Smoothes patients' transitions into and out of hospitals and other institutions
	Communicates with patients and caregivers by phone, monitoring their status regularly.
	Coaches patients in self-management.
	Facilitates patients' and caregivers' access to appropriate community services.
	Educates and supports family caregivers.

■ *Tracking the nurse's performance of essential activities* of Guided Care. The success of Guided Care depends heavily on the physician's cooperation with the nurse and the nurse's consistent performance of certain essential activities. Such activities include the expeditious establishment of the initial case load, the regular nurse's teamwork discussions with the primary care physicians and staff members, the structured monthly monitoring and coaching contacts with patients, the facilitation of transitional care, the quarterly support calls to patients' caregivers, and the discussion of advance directives with all patients. To ensure the consistent performance of these activities, the practice should operate a system of continuous quality improvement. To launch this system, the supervisor should provide the nurse with a written list of these essential activities, a performance goal (or target) for each activity (see Table 6.2), a description of how the nurse should document the performance of each activity (see Table 6.3), and a schedule of quarterly evaluation meetings at which the supervisor and

Table 6.2

PERFORMANCE TARGETS FOR GUIDED CARE NURSES

Task	Target
Orientation	
Building caseload	Two Care Guides should be created per week.
Transitional Care	
Delivering Care Guide to an inpatient professional (nurse or physician).	Care Guides should be delivered for at least 75% of all admissions within 2 days of the admission.
Preparing the patient and/or caregiver for discharge.	Discharge preparation should occur for at least 50% of all admissions within 2 days of discharge.
Post discharge in-home review of Action Plan with patient/ caregiver.	In-home reviews should occur for at least 85% of all discharges within 2 days of discharge.
Scheduled Monitoring and Coaching (SMC)	
Monitoring and coaching of patients with review of Action Plans.	At least 83% of patients should be monitored and coached each month.
Advance Directives	
Urging patients to create an Advance Directive.	Discuss Advance Directives with 100% of patients.
Caregiver Support	
Communication with patients' primary caregivers regarding needs, including: • "How are you feeling?" • "Do you need additional help?" • "Is there anything I can do to help you?" (e.g., Could a community resource help?)	At least 75% of patients' primary caregivers should be monitored once every 3 months.
Teamwork Development	
Teamwork discussions with primary care physicians.	One discussion with each physician every 2 months.

Table 6.3

DOCUMENTING ESSENTIAL ACTIVITIES OF GUIDED CARE

	ITEMS TO DOCUMENT	EXAMPLE
Transitional care	Date of admission	"1/16/09" Patient admitted to Bayview for myocardial infarction, primary care physician notified.
	Delivery of Care Guide (CG) ■ recipient of CG	"1/17/09" Handed CG to charge nurse in cardiac care unit.
	Preparation for transition ■ participant(s) ■ major topics	"1/23/09" Visited pt and caregiver in hospital; prepared them for transition home; discussed new meds, home physical therapy, Meals on Wheels.
	Date of discharge	"1/24/09" Pt discharged home, PCP notified.
	Post-discharge follow-up[a] ■ participant(s) ■ reviewed updated Action Plan (AP)	"1/25/09" Visited pt and caregiver at home; reviewed updated AP.
	Medication reconciliation[b] ■ participant(s) ■ patient taking regimen correctly	"1/25/09" Reviewed new regimen with pt and caregiver during post-discharge home visit. Pt taking regimen correctly.
Scheduled monitoring and coaching	■ topic(s) ■ follow-up plan	"2/26/09" Coached patient on limiting salt intake and using medication calendar to improve use of Lasix; she'll call me in one week to discuss progress.
	Contact attempt #1	"3/25/09" Patient did not call for scheduled monitoring and coaching (SMC).
	Contact attempt #2	"3/26/09" Attempted to call patient for SMC—no answer, left message.
	Contact attempt #3	"3/30/09 Attempted to call patient for SMC—no answer, left message.

(Continued)

Table 6.3

DOCUMENTING ESSENTIAL ACTIVITIES OF GUIDED CARE

	ITEMS TO DOCUMENT	EXAMPLE
	Letter sent	"1/31/09" Sent letter to patient
	Updated Action Plan	"1/27/09" Discovered patient has urinary incontinence; updated electronic health record and mailed new Action Plan to patient.
	Follow up on community service referral, service name	"1/26/09" Patient attending exercise classes at senior center twice/week.
Advance Directives	Discussion of Five Wishes, Durable Power of Attorney for Health Care (DPOAHC), or living will (LW) ■ topic ■ outcome ■ follow-up plan	"2/8/09" Discussed Five Wishes with patient; pt does not want to complete at this time; we'll discuss at next SMC contact.
	Advance directive completed ■ outcome ■ follow-up plan	"2/8/09" Living will completed; LW placed in medical record; Sand noted in CG and AP.

Caregiver Support

SETTING	ITEMS TO DOCUMENT	EXAMPLE
During transitional care	Post-discharge follow-up with caregiver (and pt)	"2/8/09" CAREGIVER CONTACT Visited pt and caregiver (daughter) at home to review updated Care Guide and discuss how to take new medications. Asked caregiver how she was feeling and if she needed additional help. Discussed home health service options.
Scheduled monitoring and coaching	Monitoring contact	"2/8/09" CAREGIVER CONTACT Called pt for SMC and spoke with caregiver. Reviewed Action Plan; no new meds, pt walks

(Continued)

Table 6.3

DOCUMENTING ESSENTIAL ACTIVITIES OF GUIDED CARE *(Continued)*

	ITEMS TO DOCUMENT	EXAMPLE
		daily in neighborhood with caregiver, up-to-date on screening; next PCP appt in 2 weeks.
		Asked caregiver how she was feeling and if she needed additional help.
Unscheduled call from caregiver		"2/8/09" CAREGIVER CONTACT
		Pt's daughter called today concerned about a recent fall her mother suffered.
		Asked caregiver how she was feeling and if she needed additional help.
Letter	Caregiver contact	"2/8/09" CAREGIVER CONTACT
		Dear Mrs. Smith: I am the Guided Care nurse working with your husband. I have not been able to get in touch with you recently and would like to check in with you to see how you are feeling and if you could use any additional help in caring for your husband. Please call me at your earliest convenience.

[a]Includes discharges to home or another facility. [b]This step should be done as soon as possible post-discharge.

the nurse will review and discuss the nurse's documented performance of each activity. The supervisor is responsible for the ongoing monitoring of the nurse's performance through reviews of the documentation entered by the nurse into the practice's health information technology. At the quarterly evaluation meetings, the nurse and the supervisor review the supervisor's performance reports, the nurse's self-evaluation, the nurse's assessment of the physicians' cooperation, and the staff and physician's evaluations of the nurse's performance. Nonattainment of a performance goal (e.g., delivering a Care Guide to an inpatient professional for only 50% of the hospital admissions of Guided Care patients) often helps the nurse and the supervisor to identify and resolve a system problem (e.g., the incomplete notification of the nurse when admissions occur).

Following the 6- to 8-month orientation period, during which the practice's caseload of Guided Care patients and caregivers is established, the supervisor must continue to manage many of the processes of Guided Care. Such ongoing processes include:

- Communication with insurance organizations (e.g., Medicare) that reimburse the practice for the costs of providing Guided Care for eligible patients.
- Communication with eligible patients and caregivers regarding the administrative aspects of their eligibility and enrollment in the practice's Guided Care program.
- Communication with the primary care physicians and the office staff regarding the ongoing operation and results of Guided Care within the practice.
- Communication with and supervision of the Guided Care nurse. The supervisor should meet with the Guided Care nurse regularly: (a) to assess and help improve the nurse's relationships and teamwork with the practice's physicians, office staff members, patients, and caregivers; and (b) to discuss the feedback reports regarding the nurse's attainment of the preestablished performance goals, both recently (see Table 6.4) and over time (see Figure 6.1). To create these reports, the supervisor must monitor the nurse's documentation of these activities.

Throughout this time, the Guided Care nurse is encouraged to obtain ongoing professional development and support by communicating with other Guided Care nurses and by participating in relevant professional societies, such as the National Gerontological Nursing

Table 6.4

REPORT OF GUIDED CARE NURSE'S PERFORMANCE

Transitional Care

Completion rate:

	CARE GUIDE DELIVERED TO INPATIENT PROFESSIONAL PERCENTAGE COMPLETED	DISCHARGE PREPARATION MEETING WITH PATIENT AND CAREGIVER PERCENTAGE COMPLETED	POST-DISCHARGE, IN-HOME REVIEW OF ACTION PLAN WITH PATIENT AND CAREGIVER PERCENTAGE COMPLETED
Goal[a]	75	50	85
Current quarter	82.2	42.9	92.9
Difference between current quarter, goal	+7.2	–7.1	+7.9

Timing of completed tasks:

	TIME BETWEEN ADMISSION AND CARE GUIDE DELIVERY AVERAGE NUMBER OF DAYS	TIME BETWEEN DISCHARGE PREPARATION AND DISCHARGE AVERAGE NUMBER OF DAYS	TIME BETWEEN DISCHARGE AND IN-HOME REVIEW OF ACTION PLAN AVERAGE NUMBER OF DAYS
Goal[b]	<2	<2	<2
Current quarter	1.9	1.8	2.5
Difference between current quarter, goal	+0.1 days	+0.2 days	–0.5 days

Scheduled Monitoring and Coaching

Documented sessions:

	COMPLETED PERCENTAGE	LEFT THREE MESSAGES PERCENTAGE	TOTAL PERCENTAGE
Goal	—	—	83.3
Current quarter	69.5	14.1	83.6
Difference between current quarter, goal	—	—	+0.3

(Continued)

Table 6.4

REPORT OF GUIDED CARE NURSE'S PERFORMANCE

Caregiver Contacts

	PERCENTAGE OF CAREGIVERS WITH COMPLETED CAREGIVER CONTACTS
Goal[c]	75
Current quarter	62
Difference between current quarter, goal	−13

Advance Directives
Durable Power of Attorney for Health Care (DPOAHC) or Living Will (LW).

	PERCENTAGE OF PATIENTS WITH DPOAHC OR LW RECORDED ON CARE GUIDE	PERCENTAGE OF PATIENTS WITH DISCUSSION OF DPOAHC OR LW RECORDED IN EHR	TOTAL
Goal[d]	—	—	100
End of current quarter	47.5	39.9	87.4
Difference between current total, goal	—	—	−12.6

[a]Computation excludes patients who died during hospitalization. [b]Includes transitions on weekdays (goal is 1 day) and weekends/holidays (goal is ASAP). [c]Computation: numerator is the number contacted to address caregiver issues; denominator is the number of patients with caregivers. [d]Computation: numerator is the number documented; denominator is the number of patients.

Association (www.ngna.org) and the Case Management Society of America (www.cmsa.org).

In summary, as with any successful complex process, Guided Care must be managed well. The roles and relationships of the participants must be clearly defined and understood by all. Performance must be measured and discussed. And, most important, the practice must embrace the processes of continuous quality improvement over time.

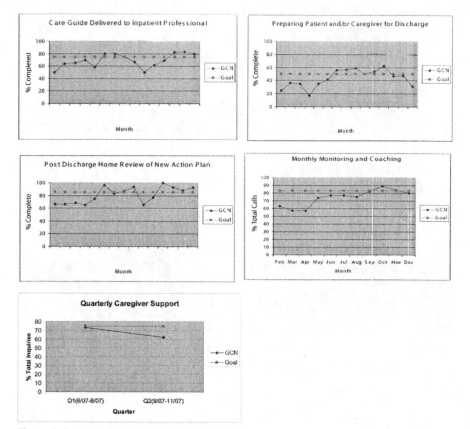

Figure 6.1 Trends in Guided Care nurses' performance.

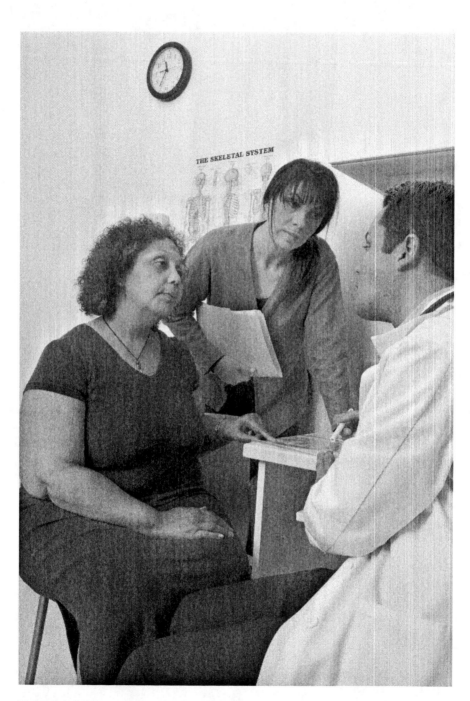

Photo 7.1 A Guided Care nurse listening to a conversation between primary care physician and Guided Care patient during an office visit.

CREDIT: Photo by Larry Canner.

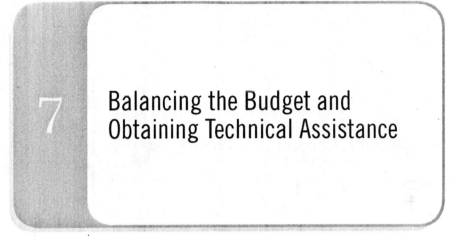

7

Balancing the Budget and Obtaining Technical Assistance

Among the physicians, nurses, patients, and caregivers who have experienced it, Guided Care is a popular method for providing high quality, effective, efficient health care for patients with chronic conditions. Rigorous studies show that, compared to "usual care," Guided Care improves physicians' satisfaction with the chronic care they provide (see Table 2.3), improves the quality of care (see Table 2.4), provides nurses with high job satisfaction, and tends to reduce the utilization and cost of health care (Boult, Reider, et al., 2008; Boyd et al., 2008; Leff et al., 2008; Sylvia et al., 2008). Yet, as described in the previous chapters, adopting Guided Care requires a practice to invest time, energy and resources in planning, launching, and operating additional services. Although many practices would like to offer Guided Care services to their chronically ill patients, few can do so without receiving supplemental funds to cover the additional costs of starting and sustaining these services.

Thus, each practice that considers adopting Guided Care must initially conduct a realistic analysis of Guided Care's likely effect on the practice's costs and revenues. The results of this analysis, combined with intangible factors such as the effects of Guided Care on staff morale and practice reputation, will inform the "business case" for (or against) adopting Guided Care. This chapter provides an approach to estimating the major costs of providing Guided Care, and it describes sources of supplemental revenue that are accessible to many practices that would like to provide Guided Care. The chapter's goal is to help leaders of practices to project the net effect of adopting Guided Care on their practice's bottom line.

THE COSTS OF PROVIDING GUIDED CARE

As shown in Table 7.1, most of the practice's additional costs for providing Guided Care result from the salary and benefits paid to the Guided Care nurse. Other costs include the nurse's equipment, communication services and local travel. In addition, the practice needs health information technology that supports Guided Care, the cost of which is highly variable. The numbers in Table 7.1 represent the actual costs incurred in studies of Guided Care in the Baltimore–Washington

Table 7.1

ANNUAL MARGINAL COSTS OF GUIDED CARE IN THE BALTIMORE METROPOLITAN AREA, 2007

	COSTS
Guided Care nurse	
Salary	$71,500[a]
Fringe benefits (at 30% of salary)	$21,450
Travel (to patients' homes, hospitals)	$588[b]
Communication services	
Internet, cell phone	$1,800
Equipment (three-year amortization)	
Computer	$500
Cell phone	$67
Total	$95,905

[a]Varies considerably by geographic area and nurse's background.
[b]*327 miles/month × 12 months × $3.00/gallon* = $588/year
            20 miles/gallon.

metropolitan areas during 2007. Some current options for practices to acquire the necessary health information technology are described in the section of chapter 4 titled Health Information Technology. The dollar values appropriate for other practices' costs will vary according to market forces in different geographic locations and practices' choices in acquiring the health information technology needed to support Guided Care.

THE REVENUE GENERATED BY GUIDED CARE

To offset the costs of providing Guided Care services, most practices need to obtain substantial additional revenues to supplement the fees they receive for providing traditional medical services through face to face physician patient encounters. Fortunately, during recent years, many organizations that pay for the health care of people with chronic conditions have acknowledged the need to provide practices with supplemental payments for chronic care services provided between patients' face-to-face encounters with physicians. Different payers require practices to provide chronically ill patients with different sets of chronic care services in order to qualify for these supplemental payments. Increasingly, practices that provide such services are being referred to by payers as "medical homes" or "patient-centered medical homes."

A practice may provide the supplemental chronic care services of a medical home—and thereby qualify for supplemental payments—in one of three ways, or a combination of these approaches. The first approach is to outsource chronic care services to a third party. The second is to redefine professional roles so that the physician(s) and the current office staff provide all of the required additional between-visit chronic care services. The third approach is to hire one or more new staff members, such as a Guided Care nurse, to provide the new services to the practice's chronically ill patients. As described starting in chapter 4, Medicare medical homes are required to use electronic health information technology, at least to track patients' chronic conditions.

In 2006, the federal Tax Relief and Health Care Act (TRHCA 06) directed the Centers for Medicare & Medicaid Services (CMS) to conduct the Medicare Medical Home Demonstration (MMHD) in eight states, beginning in 2009. During the 3 years of the demonstration, CMS will pay to each participating medical home (recognized on the basis of the chronic care services it provides) a monthly care management fee for each of its patients who is a chronically ill Medicare beneficiary. Most practices that adopt Guided Care and supportive health information technology will be capable of providing beneficiaries who have several chronic conditions with all the chronic care services CMS requires of medical homes. Those practices that participate in the MMHD will receive CMS's supplemental care management fees and shared savings payments, as well as traditional fee-for-service payments for physician–patient encounters. If the demonstration confirms that medical homes improve life for chronically ill beneficiaries and help contain the costs of the Medicare program, CMS may extend its medical home program and payments to qualified practices in all 50 states.

Private insurers, state Medicaid programs, and large employer groups are funding similar demonstration projects around the country, some which are listed in Appendix D of "A Purchaser's Guide for the Patient-Centered Medical Home" at www.pcpcc.net/content/purchaser-guide. Depending on the unique requirements of each demonstration, practices that provide Guided Care may qualify to participate and receive supplemental care management fees in these demonstrations too.

OPPORTUNITIES TO OBTAIN REVENUES TO OFFSET THE COSTS OF GUIDED CARE

In 2009, the best opportunity for a practice to obtain the supplemental revenue necessary to offset the costs of providing Guided Care is to participate in one of the current demonstrations of the medical home. The remainder of this chapter provides the details about the MMHD that were publicly available at the time this book went to press. More recently released information about this demonstration is available on the CMS Web site (www.cms.hhs.gov/DemoProjectsEvalRpts/MD/list.asp#TopofPage). Recent information about other demonstrations of the medical home is available from the organizations conducting those demonstrations (www.pcpcc.net/content/purchaser-guide).

The U.S. Congress included the MMHD in its 2006 TRHCA to help improve the quality, effectiveness, and efficiency of health care for high-need older Americans with several chronic conditions. The law requires CMS to conduct this demonstration in large and small medical homes in eight states, to pay the participating practices a monthly care management fee for each eligible beneficiary treated, and to return to the practices 80% of any net cost savings for the Medicare program. Having obtained recommendations from its "demonstration design contractor" (Mathematica Policy Research, Inc.) and several professional societies, CMS articulated the concepts listed below to operationalize this demonstration. Additional details are provided in Appendix D. CMS has also contracted with Thomson Reuters, Inc., to help implement the demonstration and with RTI International to evaluate the effects of the medical homes in the demonstration.

Design of the Demonstration

In early 2009, primary care and specialty practices in designated geographic regions of eight states will be invited (by Thomson Reuters) to apply to participate in the demonstration and, if selected by CMS, to seek recognition as medical homes. Selected practices that meet CMS's preestablished criteria for recognition as medical homes will contract with CMS to offer a defined set of chronic care services to their chronically ill Medicare beneficiaries who are eligible for the demonstration. At the end of the demonstration, the outcomes of beneficiaries who have received medical home services will be compared (by RTI) to the outcomes of similar beneficiaries who have received their health care from nonparticipating practices in the eight states. The evaluation will focus primarily on the beneficiaries' use and cost of Medicare-covered health services, but it will also assess the effects of medical homes on participating practices and on beneficiaries' health and quality of care.

Recognition as a Medical Home

To participate in the demonstration, a practice must become recognized as a "Tier 1" or "Tier 2" medical home. The services required for such recognition are listed in Appendix D, Table D.1. To obtain recognition as a medical home, a practice must describe the services it provides, and it must submit documentation of providing them to the National Committee for Quality Assurance (NCQA). Based on this information, NCQA will recognize each qualified practice as a Tier 1 or Tier 2 practice.

TransforMED (www.transformed.com) and other organizations are available to assist practices in assessing their current adherence to these

MMHD standards and in expanding their services to acquire NCQA recognition as medical homes.

Eligibility of Beneficiaries

To be eligible to participate in the demonstration, a patient must have received care from a participating medical home within the previous year, be enrolled in Medicare (Parts A and B), give informed consent to the practice, and have one or more of the chronic conditions listed in Appendix D, Resource D.1, as reported on a Medicare insurance claim during the previous 12 months. Participating beneficiaries may not be enrolled in Medicare's hospice, end stage renal disease, or Medicare Advantage programs, and they may not be long-term residents of nursing homes.

Care Management Fees

During the demonstration, CMS will pay each participating medical home a monthly care management fee for each participating beneficiary in its panel of patients. The following information was current when this book went to press, but it is subject to revision by CMS before the beginning of the demonstration. Please see www.cms.hhs.gov/DemoProjects EvalRpts/MD/list.asp#TopOfPage for updates. The amount of the fee per beneficiary depends on the tier of the participating medical home (i.e., Tier 1 or Tier 2) and the risk status of the participating beneficiary. Each beneficiary's risk of using health services heavily during the coming year is quantified as a hierarchical condition category (HCC) score. CMS uses the HCC predictive model and information from Medicare claims for the beneficiary's care during the previous year to compute each beneficiary's HCC score for the coming year (Centers for Medicare & Medicaid Services, 2008; Pope et al., 2004). Care management fees will probably average about $9,700 per month for typical Tier 1 medical homes and about $12,400 per month for typical Tier 2 medical homes. Thus, a typical Tier 2 practice that cared for 240 eligible Medicare beneficiaries could expect to receive care management fees totaling about $149,000 per year during the demonstration. These fees would offset the costs of providing Guided Care services for 60 of the practice's high-risk beneficiaries (i.e., about $96,000 per year, see Table 7.1), less intensive chronic care services for 180 of its low-risk beneficiaries (i.e., about $27,000 per year) and HIT services for all patients (i.e., about $13,000 per year) as shown in Appendix D, Table D.3).

Timeline for the Demonstration

Based on the information that was available when this book went to press, the major milestones of the demonstration are:

- January 2009: Thomson Reuters (CMS's implementation contractor) invites practices in eight states to participate in the demonstration.
- March–May 2009: Practices apply to participate; CMS selects practices to seek recognition as medical homes.
- June–November 2009: Selected practices seek recognition by the NCQA as medical homes. As applicant practices receive recognition as medical homes and execute contracts with CMS, they begin enrolling beneficiaries who are eligible and have given consent to participate in the demonstration.
- January 2010–December 2012: The demonstration is conducted.
- December 2012: The demonstration and the payment of care management fees end. RTI completes its collection of clinical data about practices and beneficiaries in the medical home and comparison groups.
- December 2013: The evaluation of the demonstration is completed.

In summary, implementing Guided Care incurs significant costs for a practice, costs that must be covered by new supplemental revenues. Fortunately, such revenues are available to practices that participate in demonstrations of the medical home that are now being sponsored by CMS and other payers for health care services. Practices that wish to transform their care of patients with chronic conditions can do so by adopting Guided Care en route to being recognized as medical homes and qualifying for supplemental care management fees that offset the costs of the transformation.

FINDING AND OBTAINING TECHNICAL ASSISTANCE

Implementing a good idea that has worked in other practices is an exciting process, but it is not a simple or easy one. Even after reading published scientific articles and instruction manuals (like this book), some practice leaders may doubt that they could adopt Guided Care successfully on their own. They fear, not inappropriately, that unforeseen obstacles may arise to slow their progress or cause the adoption to fail. Cautious practice leaders want to know that expert assistance is available to see them through the challenges of transforming their practices.

Fortunately, because of the nation's growing awareness of the need to improve chronic care, many private and public leaders are now promoting the testing of models like Guided Care and the medical home. For the hundreds of practices participating in the Medicare Medical Home Demonstration, CMS will facilitate access to several forms of educational and technical assistance. Practices that participate in this demonstration, or in other similar demonstrations sponsored by private insurers, employers, or by state Medicaid agencies (see Appendix D of "A Purchaser's Guide for the Patient-Centered Medical Home" at www. pcpcc.net/content/purchaser-guide) may obtain a wide array of such assistance, at little or no cost from not-for-profit organizations or at higher cost from for-profit consultants.

The following pages describe various types of educational and technical assistance and guidance made available by the Roger C. Lipitz Center at the Johns Hopkins Bloomberg School of Public health and its partner organizations for practices that wish to adopt Guided Care. Some of this assistance is also helpful to practices that wish to become medical homes without adopting the Guided Care model.

ONLINE COURSE FOR PHYSICIANS

The Tax Relief and Health Care Act of 2006 (Public Law 109–432) requires the personal physicians and staff members of all medical home practices to provide at least four services:

- Comprehensive, integrated, cross-disciplinary care.
- Evidence-based medicine.
- Tracking patients' health status and providing patients with convenient access to care through the use of health information technology.
- Supporting patients' management of their own conditions.

Unfortunately, most current general internal medicine (GIM) and family medicine physicians and registered nurses have not been trained to provide these chronic care services, and GIM educators report discomfort with teaching geriatrics. As a result, few traditional practices now provide these services to their multimorbid patients.

To address these deficiencies, the faculty and staff of the Lipitz Center at Johns Hopkins University drew upon their substantial knowledge, their expert consultants, and representatives of TransforMED, the American Academy of Family Physicians, the American College of Physicians, the American Geriatrics Society, and the American Board of Internal Medicine (ABIM) to create a short course that physicians can take online at their convenience. This course strengthens physicians' competencies in activities that are essential to providing high-quality comprehensive patient care in medical homes but that are rarely taught in medical school or postgraduate education. An outline of the course is located in Appendix A: Online Courses.

Building on the assumption that the physician is already an expert diagnostician and clinician, these complementary competencies include many of the skills articulated by the ABIM's 2008 Report on Comprehensive Care Internal Medicine (www.ccimreport.org/pdf/ccim-nextsteps.pdf).

This Continuing Medical Education (CME) accredited course prepares physicians to collaborate with interdisciplinary teams to provide Guided Care and other medical home services to their patients with chronic conditions. The online course is tuition-free for physicians who participate in the MMHD and is available at market rates for other physicians.

Physicians can access this online course by visiting www.medhome info.org. Those who complete this course possess important knowledge and skills that are essential to providing high-quality comprehensive chronic care. They also receive continuing medical education credits and a certificate of completion.

ONLINE COURSE FOR NURSES

This accredited course, which is offered in association with the American Nurses Association, the American Nurses Credentialing Center, the National Gerontological Nurses Association, and the Case Management Society of America, prepares registered nurses to join practices and collaborate with their physicians and office staffs to provide Guided Care to patients with chronic conditions.

Based on the original curriculum developed to train registered nurses for a randomized trial of Guided Care (Boyd et al., 2007), nursing educators at the Institute for Johns Hopkins Nursing have created a 5-week, 10 hour, online continuing education course for registered nurses who wish to practice Guided Care in nonresearch settings. An outline of the nurses' course is located in Appendix A: Online Courses. Upon successful completion of this course, nurses receive continuing nursing education credits and a Certificate in Guided Care Nursing, a credential that certifies that a nurse possesses the knowledge, skills, and abilities necessary to practice Guided Care as a member of a practice team. Nurses may apply to enroll in this course at the Institute for Johns Hopkins Nursing, www.ijhn.jhmi.edu. Tuition is waived for nurses who are employed by practices that are participating in the MMHD. Practices may encourage their current nurses to take this course, or they may preferentially hire nurses who have earned this credential.

TECHNICAL ASSISTANCE

Numerous types of technical assistance are available to practices that wish to provide Guided Care and other medical home services. Some types are accessible for no charge; others are available for fees that cover the costs of providing the assistance. Each type is described below along with contact information for obtaining it.

Descriptions of the essential features of medical homes, CMS's national MMHD, and the process by which a practice can become recognized as a medical home are available for free at medhominfo.org and through links on the Web sites of TransforMED (www.transformed.com), the Medical Group Management Association (www.mgma.com) and the American Medical Group Association (www.amga.org). These Web sites also provide links to telephone advice, answers to frequently asked questions, and other sources of assistance in becoming a medical home.

A program that allows practices to self-assess their readiness to qualify as a medical home, the Medical Home IQ tool, is available to all practices for free on the TransforMED Web site (www.transformed.com). This self-assessment program also contains links to sources of help for strengthening practices so they can become recognized as medical homes.

Health information technology is an essential tool used in Guided Care and medical homes. Such technology may be classified into two types: "local," which is software that runs on a local computer, or "distributed," which is software that is installed elsewhere and is accessed by practices through the Internet. A practice that currently has no health information technology can acquire either local or distributed technology. Practices that already use health information technology may need to enhance it to support the clinical services included in Guided Care or the medical home. Extensive information about the capabilities, performance, and prices of many commercially available electronic health record products is accessible at www.transformed.com/MedicalHome Marketplace, www.centerforhit.org, and www.acponline.org.

Some practices that wish to provide Guided Care or other medical home services may require on-site consultation by experts in these models of care. Such consultation can be obtained at market rates through TransforMED (www.transformed.com), the Medical Group Management Association (www.mgma.com) and other practice consultants.

TransforMED, in collaboration with experts in Guided Care at the Johns Hopkins Bloomberg School of Public Health, plans to conduct regional "Learning Collaboratives" in the areas in which the MMHD will occur. These workshops will assist participants in the demonstration in adopting Guided Care and becoming recognized as medical homes. More information is available at www.medhomeinfo.org.

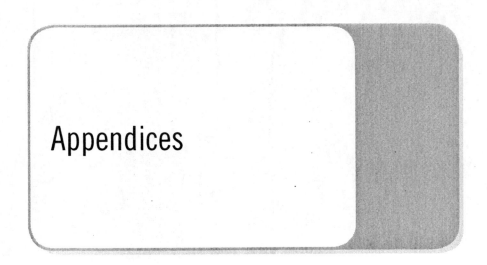

Appendices

Appendix A: Online Courses

GUIDED CARE NURSING COURSE

Most Guided Care nurses report high job satisfaction. They especially enjoy the close personal relationships they develop over time with their patients and family caregivers. Patients say, "it's like having a nurse in the family." Nurses say, "This is what I went into nursing for, to really make a difference in people's lives." Guided Care nurses also enjoy practicing in close partnership with primary care physicians, performing a wide variety of clinical tasks, and working flexible hours. One negative aspect is Guided Care nurses' occasional inability to meet all of their patients' needs on busy days, especially when several patients experience clinical deterioration simultaneously.

Many U.S. registered nurses may wish to become Guided Care nurses. About 300,000 nurses change employers each year, with increasing percentages working in ambulatory care settings and decreasing percentages working in hospitals. Furthermore, despite the national nursing shortage, approximately half a million licensed registered nurses are not currently employed in nursing, largely because of career and/or workplace issues (Health Resources and Services Administration, Bureau of Health Professions, 2004).

Although not required, certain professional experiences and characteristics are common among nurses who are especially well-suited to

145

learning and practicing Guided Care. Experience in caring for older or chronically ill patients in ambulatory settings, such as home care, hospice, or outpatient clinics, provides valuable relevant knowledge and skills. Likewise, affinity for interdisciplinary teamwork, flexibility in problem solving, strong interpersonal communication skills, and comfort with health information technology are well-suited to the practice of Guided Care.

To become recognized professionally as a Guided Care nurse, a candidate with a nursing degree and a current nursing license must complete an accredited Guided Care Nursing course and pass an examination sponsored by the American Nurses Credentialing Center of the American Nurses Association. Valid licensure to practice as a registered nurse must have been granted by a Board of Nursing of one of the 50 states.

The accredited Guided Care nursing course is only available online. It comprises 4 core units (consisting of 20 required modules and 5 live, interactive Webinars) and 17 "optional" modules. Each module consists of objectives, readings, case resources, learning activities (e.g., Power-Point lecture, assignments, and asynchronous discussion boards), self-assessment questions, and an assertion of completion. The Webinars allow the instructor and the learners to converse, demonstrate skills, and role-play in a live, online group setting.

The core units must be completed in entirety by all learners enrolled in the course, whereas completion of the optional modules is at the discretion of each individual learner. The examination, which is also taken online, tests the learners' knowledge of information covered in all 37 modules.

The four units and their required modules are:

1. "Foundations of Guided Care Nursing" unit—seven modules and one Webinar.

    Modules

    > Overview of Guided Care
    > Patient preferences for care
    > Motivational interviewing for self-management
    > Communicating with physicians
    > Assisting patients and caregivers with Medicare coverage
    > Cultural Competence
    > Overview of electronic health records

    Webinar

2. "Establishing new patients and caregivers" unit—four modules
    and one Webinar.

    Modules

    > Assessing patients' general status
    > Assessing patients' specific conditions
    > Interviewing patients' caregivers
    > Care Planning

    Webinar

3. "Ongoing Guided Care" unit—six modules, two Webinars

    Modules

    > Introduction to ongoing Guided Care
    > Monitoring and coaching
    > Accessing community resources
    > Supporting family caregivers

    Webinar

    > Coordinating providers
    > Transitional care

    Webinar

4. "Conducting Guided Care" unit—three modules, one Webinar

    Modules

    > Integration into practice
    > Teamwork
    > Boundaries

    Webinar

The elective modules provide knowledge about 17 additional specific topics that are important to Guided Care nursing. Some nurses, however, will have already acquired the necessary knowledge about some of these topics through their previous training and/or experience. Thus, nurses who believe they possess sufficient knowledge about a topic are given the option of answering the self-assessment questions associated with that module before taking the module. If their answers are correct, they need not take that module, but they are examined on the content of all 37 modules at the end of the entire course. The 17 elective modules are:

Patient education
Elder abuse

Assessment and management of 15 specific conditions:

Heart failure

Coronary artery disease

Chronic obstructive pulmonary diseased (COPD)

Hypertension

Diabetes

Dementia

Depression

Urinary incontinence

Delirium

Chronic pain

Constipation

Falls

Sleep disorders

Osteoarthritis

Osteoporosis

About 20 hours are required to complete the 20 required modules and the 5 Webinars in the 4 core units of the course. The number of additional hours depends on the number of optional modules that each individual nurse takes. The course is paced for completion in 5 weeks, followed by an online comprehensive examination. Information about registration for the course is available at www.ijhn.jhmi.edu.

After passing the online examination, the nurse receives a Certificate in Guided Care Nursing, which documents for employers, insurers, professional societies, patients, and families that the nurse possesses the knowledge, skills, and abilities needed to perform the duties of Guided Care. Nurses who do not pass the examination on their first attempt are permitted to take an alternate examination covering the same material within 3 months.

PHYSICIANS IN MEDICAL HOMES COURSE

Traditional medical education prepares physicians to diagnose and treat diseases during face-to-face encounters with patients. Reinforcing this focus on encounter-based care is the fee-for-service compensation system that pays physicians for patient visits, but not for between-visit activities such as monitoring patients' chronic conditions, answering patients' and caregivers' questions, and coordinating care with other providers. Similarly, physicians are not trained or rewarded for practicing as members of interdisciplinary teams, for promoting patient self-management, for using health information technology, or for managing systems of care or improving the quality of such systems.

Unfortunately, many innovations that improve the quality and outcomes of chronic care, including Guided Care and the medical home, depend on these skills that many physicians lack. A major challenge for the U.S. health care system, therefore, is to develop and deploy practical methods for enhancing physicians' skills in these supplemental activities.

To begin to meet this challenge, a consortium of medical educators has created a concise course for physicians in practice or in training. Supported by a grant from the John A. Hartford Foundation, this consortium included members of the American College of Physicians, the American Academy of Family Physicians, TransforMED, the American Geriatrics Society, and the American Board of Internal Medicine, as well as practicing physicians with expertise in each of the required skills. Physicians who participate in CMS's Medicare Medical Home Demonstration can take this course and earn continuing medical education credit, in whole or in part, without paying tuition. Other physicians may take the course at market rate tuition.

This course, which includes video-recorded vignettes and learner interactivity, is based on realistic case studies of physicians and practices transforming their practices. It comprises nine modules, each which has 3–5 learning objectives.

Module 1: Managing a Medical Home

1. Describe the medical home's goals for providing access to care, patient monitoring, care coordination, and population management.
2. List 4 processes that are essential to improving the quality of care in a medical home.
3. Describe 2 mechanisms for evaluating current processes in the practice.
4. Describe 4 principles of effective communicating with members of the office staff to plan and execute improvements in work processes.

Module 2: Assessing Readiness to Change (RTC) Into a Medical Home

1. Describe 3 principles for using interviews effectively to assess RTC.
2. Describe 3 principles for using surveys effectively to assess RTC.
3. Describe 3 principles for using focus groups effectively to assess RTC.
4. Describe 3 principles for using "readiness assessment data" to plan change.

Module 3: Leading Change in a Medical Home

1. Describe 3 behavioral attributes of effective medical leaders.
2. Describe 4 common pitfalls which effective leaders avoid.
3. Describe a conceptual model of gaining and using personal power and influence to promote change.
4. Describe 5 forms of individual variability in coping with and embracing change.

Module 4: Participation on Interdisciplinary Teams (IDTs) in a Medical Home

1. State 4 reasons why teamwork is important in medical homes.
2. Describe 4 attributes of effective IDTs and their members.
3. List 3 interventions that promote the development of effective IDT attributes in the medical home.
4. Identify 2 available tools for developing IDTs.

Module 5: Communicating With the Chronically Ill Patients of a Medical Home

1. Describe 3 steps of a systematic, relationship-centered approach to communicating with patients: the "ask-tell-ask" model.
2. Describe a brief method for assessing a patient's health literacy.
3. List 5 guidelines for communicating with patients by e-mail.

Module 6: Supporting Self-Management by Patients of a Medical Home

1. Define patient self-management and distinguish it from patient education.

2. Describe a 5-point strategy to help patients gain self-efficacy and change their lifestyle behaviors.
3. Describe how self-management support can be integrated into a medical home.
4. Identify 3 resources to assist patients with self-management.
5. Identify 3 resources to assist health professionals to support patients' self-management.

Module 7: Care Management in a Medical Home

1. Describe 8 goals for including a nonphysician care manager (CM) in a medical home.
2. Describe 5 tasks of a CM in developing evidence-based, patient-centered care management plans for patients with chronic conditions.
3. Describe 7 tasks of a CM in managing the care of patients with chronic conditions.
4. List 5 resources for obtaining additional information about practice-based CM.

Module 8: Continuity of Care for Patients of a Medical Home

1. Describe 5 methods to increase the continuity of patients' care in the office.
2. Describe 5 approaches to improving continuity as patients transition across other sites of care (e.g., hospitals, emergency departments, skilled nursing facilities, rehabilitation facilities).
3. Describe 9 approaches to improving the continuity of outpatient care as patients transition between primary care and specialists.
4. Describe 9 approaches to improving the continuity of outpatient care as patients transition between primary care and home care.

Module 9: Health Information Technology (HIT) in a Medical Home

1. Describe 5 medical home functions that can be performed by HIT.
2. Describe 3 processes facilitated by HIT that satisfy *requirements* for recognition as a CMS Tier 2 medical home.

3. Describe 4 ways that implementing HIT could benefit a practice.
4. List 3 resources that provide additional detailed information about selecting, implementing, and using HIT in office practice.

Methods

Physicians complete the modules and the final assessment quiz that address the module's objectives through asynchronous communication with the host Web site. Each module contains brief reading material, an audio-enhanced PowerPoint presentation, self-assessment questions, a video vignette, final assessment questions, and optional resources for further learning. Requiring 30–60 minutes to complete, each module will link to a common case study to further facilitate learners' interaction with the course.

Evaluation

At the end of each module, physicians will take an online, multiple-choice examination of his or her attainment of the course objectives. Those who pass the examination will receive a certificate and credit for completing continuing medical education.

Physicians can register for this course through www.medhomeinfo. org.

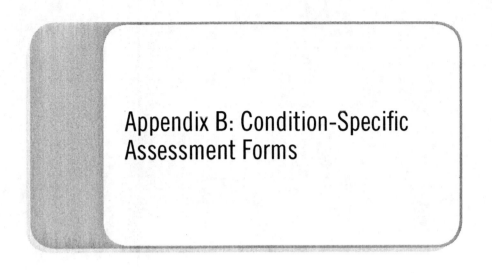

Appendix B: Condition-Specific Assessment Forms

Disability

Current management

How do you manage these activities with which you have difficulty?	Help by a person	Help by a device	Help by a service agency	Is this adequate?	
Transportation/walking outside the home	❏	❏	❏	❏ Yes	❏ No
Shopping	❏	❏	❏	❏ Yes	❏ No
Preparing meals	❏	❏	❏	❏ Yes	❏ No
Light housework	❏	❏	❏	❏ Yes	❏ No
Bathing	❏	❏	❏	❏ Yes	❏ No
Dressing	❏	❏	❏	❏ Yes	❏ No
Toileting	❏	❏	❏	❏ Yes	❏ No
Transferring	❏	❏	❏	❏ Yes	❏ No
Eating	❏	❏	❏	❏ Yes	❏ No
Walking in home	❏	❏	❏	❏ Yes	❏ No

If "not adequate," triggers suggestion for referral

<u>Potential dangers</u>   <u>Describe</u>
Physical barrier to home entry   _____
Physical barrier inside home   _____
Unsafe stove   _____

<u>Most recent consultation</u>
Physical therapist   _____/_____   ❏ Never
Occupational therapist   _____/_____   ❏ Never
Orthotist   _____/_____   ❏ Never

Previous management   **Reason for stopping or not starting**
❏ None

Device   _____   _____
Service   _____   _____
Home Modification _____   _____

Urinary Incontinence

Background

Year of onset _____

Surgery for urinary incontinence   ❏ No
                                       ❏ Yes →
                                       Suspension _____(year)
                                       Injection   _____(year)
                                       Other   _____

Cause   Severity
❏ Stress   Frequency _____ daytime episodes per week
❏ Urge   Nocturia _____ episodes per night
❏ Overflow   Amount of urine lost:
❏ Mixed   ❏ Large
❏ Unknown   ❏ Medium
❏ Other: _____   ❏ Small

Consequences
Limits fluid intake   ❏ Yes   ❏ No
Limits number of trips outside the home   ❏ Yes   ❏ No
Limits sexual activity   ❏ Yes   ❏ No

Current management
Pads   ❏ Yes   ❏ No
Scheduled voiding   ❏ Yes   ❏ No
Pelvic muscle exercises   ❏ Yes   ❏ No
Urinary catheter   ❏ Yes   ❏ No
Bladder training   ❏ Yes   ❏ No

Previous management   **Reason for stopping or not starting**
❏ None

Medicine _____   _____
Other _____   _____

Dementia

Background

History of dementia or Alzheimer's disease
❑ No
❑ Yes ➔ year of onset _____

Previous management	**Reason for stopping or not starting**
❑ None	

Medicine   _____   _____
Other   _____   _____

Falls

Background

Usual cause of falling   Injuries from falling
❑ Trip   ❑ No
❑ Dizziness   ❑ Yes _____(year) _____
❑ Balance   _____(year) _____
❑ Syncope
❑ Unknown
❑ Other: _____

Current management

Adaptive footwear
❑ None
❑ Type _____

Previous evaluation for falls
Physical therapy PT   ❑ No   ❑ Yes ➔ _____/_____ Recommendations _____
Occupational therapy OT   ❑ No   ❑ Yes ➔ _____/_____ Recommendations _____
Orthotist   ❑ No   ❑ Yes ➔ _____/_____ Recommendations _____
Podiatrist   ❑ No   ❑ Yes ➔ _____/_____ Recommendations _____
Physician   ❑ No   ❑ Yes ➔ _____/_____ Recommendations _____

Previous management   **Reason for stopping or not starting**
❑ None

Exercise for gait/balance	
Ambulatory aids	
Brace/orthosis	
Home safety modifications	
Medication	
Other	

Insomnia

Background

Year of onset _____

Pattern of sleep
❑ Difficulty falling asleep
❑ Frequently awakening
❑ Early morning awakening

Symptoms

Daytime sleepiness	❑ Yes	❑ No
Irritability	❑ Yes	❑ No
Daytime naps	❑ Yes	❑ No
Night time leg movements	❑ Yes	❑ No
Apnea/breathlessness	❑ Yes	❑ No

Contributing factors

Caffeinated beverages (coffee, tea, soft drinks): _____ per day

Any after noon?	❑ Yes	❑ No
Any after 6 p.m.?	❑ Yes	❑ No
Exercise after 6 p.m.?	❑ Yes	❑ No
Medications after 6 p.m.?	❑ Yes	❑ No

Previous management   **Reason for stopping or not starting**

❑ None

Medication _____   _____
Other   _____   _____

Osteoporosis

Background

Year of diagnosis _____

Year(s) of bone(s) or fragility fracture(s)
Year   Fracture type

_____   _____

_____   _____

_____   _____

_____   _____

Cause
❑ Postmenopausal
❑ Other: _____
❑ Not recorded

Previous management   **Reason for stopping or not starting**
❑ None

Medication _____   _____
Other   _____   _____

Diabetes

Background

Year of onset _____

Year(s) of hospital admission for diabetes _____   _____   _____

Effects

Eyes (retinopathy)	❏ Yes	❏ No
Nerves (decreased sensation in feet)	❏ Yes	❏ No
Burning night pain in feet	❏ Yes	❏ No
Kidneys (renal insufficiency)	❏ Yes	❏ No
Proteinuria or microalbuminuria	❏ Yes	❏ No

Current management

Monitoring blood sugar at home: _____ time(s) per day

Glucometer
❏ Functional
❏ Non functional
❏ N/A

Previous management   **Reason for stopping or not starting**

❏ None

Medicine   _____   _____

Other   _____   _____

Chronic Obstructive Pulmonary Disease (COPD)

Background

Year of onset _____

Most recent COPD hospital admission_____

<u>Cause</u>

❑ Smoking

❑ Other: _____

<u>Severity</u>

Dyspnea with:

❑ Stairs

❑ One-fourth block

❑ One block

❑ A few yards

❑ At rest

<u>Equipment functional</u>

Oxygen system	❑ Yes	❑ No
Nebulizer	❑ Yes	❑ No
Inhalers	❑ Yes	❑ No

Previous management   **Reason for stopping or not starting**

❑ None

Medicine   _____   _____

Other   _____   _____

Congestive Heart Failure (CHF)

Background

Year of onset _____
Most recent year of hospital admission for CHF _____
Most recent year of hospital admission for myocardial infarction (MI) _____

<u>Pacemaker</u>
❑ Yes
❑ No

<u>Cause</u>	<u>Severity of dyspnea</u>	<u>Positional effects</u>
❑ MI	❑ At rest	❑ Lying flat
❑ Valve problem	❑ Few yards	❑ Sleeping
❑ Rhythm problem	❑ 1 block	
	❑ One-fourth mile	
	❑ One flight of stairs	

<u>Equipment</u>
Scale ➔ functional   ❑ Yes   ❑ No

Current management
Monitoring weight at home: _____ time(s)/month

Previous management   **Reason for stopping or not starting**
❑ None

Medicine   _____   _____
Other   _____   _____

Coronary Artery Disease

Background

Year of onset _____

<u>Complications (if any)</u>

Year(s) of heart attack/MI _____ _____ _____

Year(s) of CABG/stent   _____ _____ _____

Year of onset of CHF   _____

<u>Symptoms</u>	Frequency
Chest discomfort	❏ Daily
❏ At rest	❏ Few days
❏ Slow walking	❏ Week
❏ Brisk walking	❏ Few weeks
❏ Climbing stairs	❏ Month
❏ With emotion	❏ Few months
	❏ Rarely

Previous management   **Reason for stopping or not starting**

❏ None

Medicine   _____   _____

Other   _____   _____

Constipation

Background

Year of onset _____

Severity

Straining _____ times per week

Incomplete evacuation _____ times per week

Abdominal bloating _____ times per week

Pattern of bowel movement

Frequency: _____ BMs per week

Typical consistency
❑ Hard
❑ Soft
❑ Liquid

Current management

Daily oral hydration
❑ <16 oz.
❑ 17–31 oz.
❑ 32+ oz.

Previous management   **Reason for stopping or not starting**

❑ None

Medicine _____   _____
Other   _____   _____

Depression

Background

History of depression
❑ Yes → Year of onset _____
❑ No

Suicidal activity
❑ No
❑ Yes → Year _____

Recent losses or crises
❑ None
❑ Yes → Describe

_____
_____
_____
_____

Previous management   **Reason for stopping or not starting**
❑ None

Medicine   _____   _____
Counseling _____   _____
Electroconvulsive therapy (ECT)
                   _____   _____
Other   _____   _____

Osteoarthritis

Background

Year of onset _____

Area(s) most affected
❏ Hip
❏ Knee
❏ Hand
❏ Wrist
❏ Shoulder
❏ Spine
❏ Neck
❏ Foot
❏ Ankle
❏ Elbow

Functional limitation by arthritis
❏ None
❏ A little
❏ A lot

Previous management
❏ None

Medicine _____
PT/OT _____
Orthopedic consultation _____
Other _____

Reason for stopping or not starting

_____
_____
_____
_____

Persistent Pain

Background

Year of onset _____

Description of pain
- ❑ Discomfort
- ❑ Soreness
- ❑ Hurting
- ❑ Aching

Location(s) most affected
- ❑ Hip
- ❑ Knee
- ❑ Back
- ❑ Neck
- ❑ Foot
- ❑ Head
- ❑ Abdomen
- ❑ Other: _____

Cause
- ❑ Arthritis
- ❑ Diabetes
- ❑ Cancer
- ❑ Other: _____

Pain limits
- ❑ Daily activities
- ❑ Social activities
- ❑ Quality of life

Current management

Physical treatments
- ❑ Heat
- ❑ Cold
- ❑ Acupuncture
- ❑ Pressure
- ❑ Transcutaneous electrical nerve stimulation (TENS)
- ❑ Salve
- ❑ Massage
- ❑ Chiropractor

Previous management

- ❑ None

Medicine _____
Physical treatments _____
Other: _____

Reason for stopping or not starting

_____

_____

_____

Hypertension

Background

Year of onset

Year(s) of hospital admission for BP

Year(s) of hospital admission for CHF

Year(s) of heart attack

Year(s) of stroke

Current management

Home BP _____ times per month

Community BP _____ times per month

<u>BP device</u>

❏ Functional

❏ Non-functional

Previous management

❏ None

Medicine _____

Other _____

Reason for stopping or not starting

_____

_____

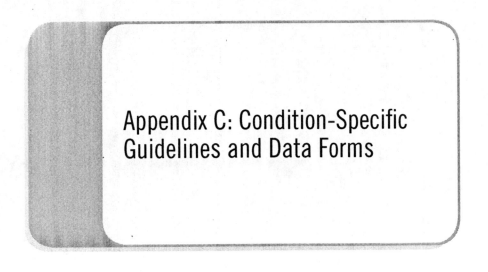

Appendix C: Condition-Specific Guidelines and Data Forms

Angina

Guidelines

Diet
Low-fat

Education
Smoking cessation

Medications
All CAD patients: Aspirin, B-blocker
CAD patients with angina: NTG (SL or nasal spray), ACE- inhibitor, long-acting nitrates, long-acting Ca-blockers
CAD patients with any elevation in LDL: statin

Monitoring
Annual visit to physician with lipid profile and LFTs if taking a statin

Physical activity
Regular mild–moderate exercise

Targets

Red flags

Background information

Year of onset
Year of onset of CHF

More recent results

Measure	Date	Results

You are required to ensure that your request
for data is consistent with the HIPAA policy   Name:
on minimum necessary uses and disclosures   DOB:

Congestive Heart Failure (CHF)

Guidelines

Diet
Sodium restriction

Medications
Avoid: NSAIDS, Ca channel blockers (if low EF)
Diuretics, ACEI/ARB, B-blockers, aldosterone inhibitor, digitalis, vasodilators

Monitoring
Daily weights
Monitor K

Other
Avoid: tobacco, alcohol

Physical activity
Regular mild–moderate exercise

Targets

Red flags

Background information
Year of onset

Most recent results

Measure	Date	Results

You are required to ensure that your request
for data is consistent with the HIPAA policy
on minimum necessary uses and disclosures

Name:
DOB:

Chronic Obstructive Pulmonary Disease (COPD)/Asthma

Guidelines

Education
Smoking cessation
Use of inhalers

Medications
Primary: long-acting bronchodilators—inhaled B2-agonists and/or anticholinergics and/or oral theophylline
Secondary: inhaled steroids, oxygen

Physical activity
Regular mild–moderate exercise

Referral
Pulmonary rehabilitation

Targets

Red flags

Background information

Year of onset

Most recent results

Measure	Date	Results

You are required to ensure that your request
for data is consistent with the HIPAA policy   Name:
on minimum necessary uses and disclosures   DOB:

Dementia

Guidelines

Medications

Avoid: sedative, opioid, anticholinergic

Consider potential benefits, risks, and costs of cholinesterase inhibitor for mild–moderate Alzheimer's disease

Other

Information and support for caregiver(s) for dementia

Remove exposure to contributing factors: medications, alcohol

Physical activity

Regular mild–moderate exercise

Targets

Red flags

Background information

Year of onset

Most recent results

Measure	Date	Results

You are required to ensure that your request
for data is consistent with the HIPAA policy   Name:
on minimum necessary uses and disclosures   DOB:

Diabetes

Guidelines

Medications

Hypoglycemic agent(s), ASA (75 mg/day), ACEI/ARB (if + proteinuria), statin (if LDL > 100), antihypertensive (if BP > 130/80)

Monitoring

Annual microalbumin, creatinine, K, LDL (or more frequently, as needed)
Daily fingerstick glucose (if on insulin) by patient or caregiver
Daily foot inspection (if sensory neuropathy is present) by patient or caregiver
HgA1c every 6 months (or more frequently, as needed)

Other

Monitoring by primary care physician foot exam, BP at each office visit

Physical activity

Moderate aerobic exercise 30–45 minutes 3–5 days per week

Referral

Medical nutrition therapy (MNT) per certified diabetes educator (CDE)

Specialist

Annual dilated retinal exam by ophthalmologist

Targets

Red flags

Background information

Year of onset

Most recent results

Measure	Date	Results

Falling

Guidelines

Education
Educate patient and caregiver about preventing falls

Other
Appropriate use of ambulation aids
Correction/modification of intrinsic risks: visual deficits, foot problems, joint problems, neurologic disorders, muscle weakness, orthostasis, and cardiac dysrhythmias
Multifactorial evaluation to determine the cause(s) of falling
Remove or modify exposure to extrinsic risks: psychotropic medications, environmental hazards, improper footwear

Physical activity
Gait, strength and balance training

Targets

Red flags

Background information

Year of onset

Most recent results

Measure	Date	Results

Name:
DOB:

Hypertension

Guidelines

Diet
Sodium restriction

Medication
Diuretic, beta-blocker, ACEI/ARB, CCB

Monitoring
Monitor blood pressure monthly (if within target range)

Physical Activity
Regular mild–moderate exercise

Targets

Red flags

Background information

Year of onset

Most recent results

Measure	Data	Results

You are required to ensure that your request
for data is consistent with the HIPAA policy   Name:
on minimum necessary uses and disclosures   DOB:

Insomnia

Guidelines

Diet
Avoid: alcohol, caffeinated coffee, tea, soft drinks, and chocolate

Medications
Avoid long-term use of hypnotics and sedatives
Avoid: sympathomimetics, bronchodilators, and diuretics after 6 p.m.

Monitoring
Maintain a sleep diary

Physical activity
Daily mild–moderate exercise, none after 6 p.m.

Referral
Seek cause of insomnia: pain, voiding, depression, anxiety, caffeine, stimulant medicine, alcohol, GERD, restless legs syndrome, sleep apnea

Targets

Red flags

Background information
Year of onset

Most recent results

Measure	Date	Results

You are required to ensure that your request
for data is consistent with the HIPAA policy   Name:
on minimum necessary uses and disclosures   DOB:

Osteoporosis

Guidelines

Diet

Ingest dairy products and supplements that provide at least 1,200 mg/day of calcium and 800 IU/day of vitamin D

Education

Do not smoke or use alcohol excessively

Medications

Avoid: corticosteroids

Take bisphosphonate, calcitonin

Monitoring

Central BMD scan every 2 years

Physical activity

Daily weight-bearing or resistance exercise

Targets

Red flags

Background information

Year of onset

Most recent results

Measure	Date	Results

You are required to ensure that your request
for data is consistent with the HIPAA policy   Name:
on minimum necessary uses and disclosures   DOB:

Urinary Incontinence

Guidelines

Diet

Avoid: caffeine, alcohol, and evening fluid intake

Prevent dehydration: ensure intake of 32+ fluid oz daily

Medications

Avoid: diuretics, b-blockers, anticholinergics (in some cases)

Monitoring

Complete bladder diary

Evaluation: history, bladder diary, physical/pelvic exam, urinalysis, PVR

Other

Minimize leakage: absorbent padding

Minimize leakage: ensure easy access to toilet or commode

Minimize leakage: scheduled voiding

Prevent skin breakdown: cleanse after each incontinent episode

Targets

Red flags

Background information

Year of onset

Most recent results

Measure	Date	Results

Name:

DOB:

Appendix D: Centers for Medicare & Medicaid Services' Medicare Medical Home Demonstration (MMHD)

The Medicare Medical Home Demonstration (MMHD) provides an excellent opportunity for a national evaluation of the effects of several new models of improved chronic care for older Americans. Guided Care is one such model; other models will be tested as well. To understand how Guided Care and other models could provide medical home services and, thereby, qualify for participation in CMS's MMHD, one must know the details about how the MMHD will be conducted. For example, how does CMS define a medical home? How can a practice obtain CMS recognition as a medical home? What will be the amounts of the supplemental care management payments and shared savings payments, in addition to the usual encounter-based fee-for-service payments' that CMS will make to participating practices? Which patients will qualify to receive medical home services (and thereby generate supplemental payments to the practice)?

Practices that are considering participation in the MMHD would be wise to consider what may happen after the demonstration ends in 2012. Will CMS continue to provide care management fees to all medical home practices, or only to the types of practices that succeeded in reducing Medicare's costs during the demonstration? Will practice types that did not reduce Medicare expenditures lose access to care management fees in the future?

This appendix provides answers to many of these questions. The information provided here was current when this book went to press. Readers are cautioned, however, that CMS's plans for conducting the demonstration continued to evolve into 2009. During this dynamic time, strong political forces actively attempted to shape the implementation and evaluation of the MMHD and the postdemonstration funding of medical homes. Up-to-date information about these issues is available at the CMS Web site (www.cms.hhs.gov/DemoProjectsEvalRpts/MD/list.asp) and www.medhomeinfo.org and through the sources of technical assistance described in chapter 7, for example, the Web sites of TransforMED (www.transformed.com), the Medical Group Management Association (www.mgma.com), the American College of Physicians (www.acponline.org), and the American Medical Group Association (www.amga.org).

THE HISTORY OF THE MEDICARE MEDICAL HOME DEMONSTRATION

In December 2006, the U.S. Congress passed and President George W. Bush signed into law the Tax Relief and Health Care Act (TRHCA), which directed CMS to conduct the MMHD. In September 2007, CMS awarded a contract to Mathematica Policy Research (MPR) to recommend a design for the demonstration. MPR submitted its preliminary recommendations in early 2008 and its final recommendations to CMS in mid-2008. In July 2008, the U.S. Congress overrode a presidential veto to pass Public Law 110-275, which provides an additional $100 million for expanding the demonstration and continuing payments to medical homes after 2012.

This appendix contains CMS's initial plans for conducting the demonstration. These plans may undergo revision by CMS during early 2009, however, so the final details of the operation of the demonstration may not be known until spring 2009 or later. In addition to the TransforMED, Medical Group Management Association, and American Group Management Association Web sites, up-to-date information is accessible on the CMS Web site (www.cms.hhs.gov/DemoProjectsEvalRpts/MD/list.asp).

OVERVIEW

The Centers for Medicare and Medicaid Services (CMS) will conduct the medical home demonstration as directed by Section 204 of the TRHCA of 2006. The act calls for the project to provide targeted, accessible, continuous, and coordinated family centered care to high-need populations through a medical home demonstration. The act also specifies that the demonstration will include Medicare beneficiaries who are deemed to be "high need" (i.e., with multiple chronic conditions or prolonged illnesses that require regular medical monitoring, advising, or treatment). The MMHD will be conducted in up to eight states, including urban, rural, and underserved areas, over a 3-year period. CMS planned to announce the MMHD locales in early 2009.

According to Section 204 of the TRHCA, a "medical home" is a physician practice that is responsible for targeted, accessible, continuous, coordinated, family-centered care to high-need populations. Care is provided by a "personal physician" who is assigned to an individual patient participant. The responsibilities of a medical home also include targeting beneficiaries for participation in the demonstration and providing safe and secure technology to promote patient access to personal health information. In addition, a medical home is responsible for developing a health assessment tool for beneficiary participants and for providing training programs for staff involved in the coordination of care. To qualify as a medical home, a large or small physician practice must employ board-certified physicians. Practices may employ primary care, specialty, or subspecialty physicians, such as cardiologists and oncologists.

ELIGIBILITY OF PRACTICES TO PARTICIPATE IN THE DEMONSTRATION

To be recognized as a medical home, a practice must document having specific core capabilities that enable the personal physician to coordinate all of the patient's medical care. Participating practices must submit their capabilities with documentation in a process referred to as "recognition." Each practice's capabilities are reviewed and evaluated to determine if they meet the core capability requirements to become a medical home. The recognition process is similar to that used by the National Committee for Quality Assurance's Physician Practice Connections®—Patient-Centered Medical Home™ (PPC-PCMH™) program.

In this demonstration, CMS will recognize each participating practice as a medical home in a specific tier. "Tier 1" medical homes are considered "basic" homes. "Tier 2" contains "advanced" medical homes that are capable of providing all medical home services.

In all participating medical homes, the personal physician must provide the following functions or services:

- Advocates for and provides ongoing support, oversight and guidance to implement a plan of care that provides integrated, coherent, cross-disciplinary care in partnership with beneficiary participants and all other physicians furnishing care to the beneficiary participant.
- Uses evidence-based medicine and evidence-based clinical support tools to guide decision making at the point-of-care.
- Uses health information technology (HIT) that may include remote monitoring and patient registries to monitor and track the health status of beneficiary participants.
- Provides enhanced and convenient access to health care for beneficiary participants.

The Application Process

The process for practices to apply to participate in the demonstration, including the application form and instructions, will be made available to practices electronically and in printed form. CMS envisions a recruitment goal of 50 practices in each of eight locales with up to 2,000 physicians in total.

CMS will evaluate each application for eligibility according to seven criteria:

- Is a physician-based practice in primary care or a specialty or subspecialty that also provides primary care services. This will include Federally Qualified Health Centers (FQHC) and Community Health Centers (CHC).
- Is staffed by board-certified physicians who will perform the services of a personal physician.
- Provides the majority of primary health care to their eligible patients.
- Possesses a valid and current Medicare National Provider Identification (NPI) number.
- Agrees to perform medical home services as described by CMS in one of the medical home tiers.
- Agrees to participate for the duration of the demonstration.
- Sees an average of 150 or more Medicare beneficiaries in practice.

The application period for the demonstration is scheduled to begin in March 2009, and continue through May, 2009.

The Medical Home Recognition Process

The Centers for Medicare & Medicaid Services will conduct a procedure for practices with approved applications to become recognized as medical homes. CMS will provide approved physician practices with the criteria for recognition, provide instructions for submission of practice capabilities and documentation, and provide customer service and limited technical assistance to practices throughout the recognition procedure. There are two medical home tiers.

- Tier 1 is considered a basic medical home that possesses capabilities sufficient to provide basic care coordination services to participating beneficiaries.
- Tier 2 is an advanced medical home that is capable of providing the highest level of care coordination, using an electronic health record to manage patient needs.

Practices will identify their medical home capabilities through the completion of a self-attestation survey tool followed by the submission of supporting documentation that NCQA will use to determine whether to recognize them in Tier 1 or Tier 2. This process will be similar to one used by NCQA to recognize medical home practices under the PPC-PCMH™ model. The NCQA estimates that the self-attestation survey can be completed in 2 to 4 hours, while gathering the necessary documentation could take 2 to 3 months. The NCQA reports being able to complete the review of completed recognition packages (assuming all the pieces are together) within 30 days. CMS's criteria for recognition as a medical home appear in Table D.1.

Assistance With the Recognition Process

The Centers for Medicare & Medicaid Services will develop a training program to assist practices in submitting the information on which they hope to be recognized as medical homes. CMS does not envision providing guidance in becoming a medical home, but simply to assist practices in completing the recognition process. Therefore, training sessions will be conducted at a high level and geared toward physicians and practice administrators, to provide guidance in submitting the self-attestation and supporting documentation for recognition as a medical home.

Table D.1

DEFINITIONS OF MEDICAL HOME TIERS

TIER 1	TIER 2
ALL 17 OF THE FOLLOWING REQUIREMENTS (17 CORE)	**ALL 19 OF THE FOLLOWING REQUIREMENTS** / **THREE OF THE 9 ADDITIONAL REQUIREMENTS**

CONTINUITY

1. The practice discusses with patients and presents written information on the role of the medical home that addresses up to 8 areas.	1. The practice discusses with patients and presents written information on the role of the medical home that addresses up to 8 areas.
2. The practice establishes written standards on scheduling each patient with a personal clinician for continuity of care and the practice collects data to show that it meets its standards on continuity.	2. The practice establishes written standards on scheduling each patient with a personal clinician for continuity of care and the practice collects data to show that it meets its standards on continuity.

CLINICAL INFORMATION SYSTEMS

3. The practice uses an electronic data system that includes searchable data such as patient demographics, visit dates and diagnoses (up to 12 specific factors), and the practice uses an electronic or paper-based system to identify clinically important conditions or risk factors among its patient population.	3. The practice uses an electronic data system that includes searchable data such as patient demographics, visit dates and diagnoses (up to 12 specific factors), and the practice uses an electronic or paper-based system to identify clinically important conditions or risk factors among its patient population, and the practice has an electronic health record, certified by the Certification Commission on Health Information Technology (C-CHIT), that
	20. The practice uses an electronic system to write prescriptions which can print or send prescriptions electronically, clinicians in the practice write prescriptions using electronic prescription reference information at the point of care, which includes safety alerts that may be generic or specific to the patient (up to 8 specific factors), and clinicians engage in cost-efficient prescribing by using a prescription writer that has general automatic alerts for

generic options or is connected to a payer-specific formulary.

21. The practice provides patients/families with access to an interactive Web site that allows electronic communication.

22. The practice provides for patient access to personal health information such as test results or prescription refills or to see elements of their medical record and import elements of their medical record into a personal health record.

DELIVERY SYSTEM REDESIGN

23. The practice measures or receives data on performance such as clinical process, clinical outcomes, service data or patient safety issues, and the practice collects data on patient experience with care, addressing up to 3 areas.

24. The practice reports performance data to physicians.

25. The practice uses performance data to set goals and take action where identified to improve performance.

captures searchable data on clinical information such as blood pressure, lab results or status of preventive services (up to 9 specific areas).

4. The practice establishes written standards to support patient access, including policies for scheduling visits and responding to telephone calls and electronic communication (up to 9 specific factors).

5. The practice collects data to demonstrate that it meets standards related to appointment scheduling and response times for telephone and electronic communication (up to 5 specific factors).

4. The practice establishes written standards to support patient access, including policies for scheduling visits and responding to telephone calls and electronic communication (up to 9 specific factors).

5. The practice collects data to demonstrate that it meets standards related to appointment scheduling and response times for telephone and electronic communication (up to 5 specific factors).

(Continued)

DEFINITIONS OF MEDICAL HOME TIERS *(Continued)*

TIER 1 ALL 17 OF THE FOLLOWING REQUIREMENTS (17 CORE)	TIER 2 ALL 19 OF THE FOLLOWING REQUIREMENTS	THREE OF THE 9 ADDITIONAL REQUIREMENTS
6. The practice defines roles for physician and non-physician staff and trains staff, with non-physician staff, involved in reminding patients of appointments, executing standing orders and educating patients/families.	6. The practice defines roles for physician and non-physician staff and trains staff, with non-physician staff, involved in reminding patients of appointments, executing standing orders and educating patients/families.	26. The practice uses electronic information to generate lists of patients and take action to remind patients or clinicians proactively of services needed, such as patients needing clinician review or action or reminders for preventive care, specific tests or follow-up visits (up to 5 specific factors).
7. The practice uses electronic or paper-based tools including medication lists and other tools such as problem lists, or structured templates for notes or preventive services to organize and document clinical information in the medical record.	7. The practice uses electronic or paper-based tools including medication lists and other tools such as problem lists, or structured templates for notes or preventive services to organize and document clinical information in the medical record.	27. The practice uses a paper-based or electronic system for reminders at the point of care based on guidelines for preventive services such as screening tests, immunizations, risk assessments and counseling.
8. The practice conducts a comprehensive health assessment for all new patients to understand their risks and needs including past medical history, risk factors and preferences for advance care planning (up to 5 specific factors).	8. The practice conducts a comprehensive health assessment for all new patients to understand their risks and needs including past medical history, risk factors and preferences for advance care planning (up to 5 specific factors).	28. The practice uses a paper-based or electronic system for reminders at the point of care based on guidelines for chronic care needs.
9. For three clinically important conditions, the physician and non-physician staff conduct care management	9. For three clinically important conditions, the physician and non-physician staff conduct care management	

using an integrated care plan to set goals, assess progress and address barriers (5 specific factors).

10. For three clinically important conditions, the physician and non-physician staff conduct care management planning ahead of the visit to make sure that information is available and the staff is prepared as well as following up after the visit to make sure that the treatment plan (including medications, tests, referrals) is implemented.

11. The practice identifies appropriate evidence-based guidelines that are used as the basis of care for clinically important conditions.

PATIENT/FAMILY ENGAGEMENT

12. The practice supports patient/family self-management through activities such as systematically assessing patient/family-specific communication barriers and preferences, providing self-monitoring tools or personal health record, and providing a written care plan.

13. The practice supports patient/family self-management through providing educational resources, and providing/connecting families to self-management resources.

using an integrated care plan to set goals, assess progress and address barriers (5 specific factors).

10. For three clinically important conditions, the physician and non-physician staff conduct care management planning ahead of the visit to make sure that information is available and the staff is prepared as well as following up after the visit to make sure that the treatment plan (including medications, tests, referrals) is implemented.

11. The practice identifies appropriate evidence-based guidelines that are used as the basis of care for clinically important conditions.

PATIENT/FAMILY ENGAGEMENT

12. The practice supports patient/family self-management through activities such as systematically assessing patient/family-specific communication barriers and preferences, providing self-monitoring tools or personal health record, and providing a written care plan.

13. The practice supports patient/family self-management through providing educational resources, and providing/connecting families to self-management resources.

(Continued)

DEFINITIONS OF MEDICAL HOME TIERS *(Continued)*

TIER 1 ALL 17 OF THE FOLLOWING REQUIREMENTS (17 CORE)	TIER 2 ALL 19 OF THE FOLLOWING REQUIREMENTS	THREE OF THE 9 ADDITIONAL REQUIREMENTS
14. The practice encourages family involvement in all aspects of patient self-management.	14. The practice encourages family involvement in all aspects of patient self-management.	

COORDINATION

15. The practice systematically tracks tests and follows up using steps such as making sure that results are available to the clinician, flagging abnormal test results, and following up with patients/families on all abnormal test results (up to 4 specific factors).	15. The practice systematically tracks tests and follows up using steps such as making sure that results are available to the clinician, flagging abnormal test results, and following up with patients/families on all abnormal test results (up to 4 specific factors).	
16. The practice coordinates referrals designated as critical through steps such as providing the patient and referring physician with the reason for the consultation and pertinent clinical findings, tracking the status of the referral, obtaining a report back from the practitioner, and asking patients about self-referrals and obtaining reports from the practitioner(s).	16. The practice coordinates referrals designated as critical through steps such as providing the patient and referring physician with the reason for the consultation and pertinent clinical findings, tracking the status of the referral, obtaining a report back from the practitioner, and asking patients about self-referrals and obtaining reports from the practitioner(s).	

17. The practice reviews all medications
    a patient is taking including
    prescriptions, over the counter
    medications and herbal therapies/
    supplements.

17. The practice reviews all medications
    a patient is taking including
    prescriptions, over the counter
    medications and herbal therapies/
    supplements.

18. The practice on its own or in conjunction
    with an external organization has a
    systematic approach for identifying and
    coordinating care for patients who receive
    care in inpatient or outpatient facilities
    or patients who are transitioning to other
    care (up to 6 specific factors).

19. The practices reviews post-hospitalization
    medication lists and reconciles with other
    medications.

CMS will accept for the demonstration only practices that are recognized as Tier 1 or Tier 2. CMS may also limit the number of participating practices to achieve a desired distribution of practices across the tiers of medical homes and across the demonstration locales.

Within 2 weeks of the end date for submitting applications, CMS will identify physician practices that are eligible for the demonstration and send letters of approval or denial to all practices that applied for the demonstration. The anticipated recognition period will be from June 2009 through November 2009, thereby allowing the demonstration to begin in January 2010. If an insufficient number of practices have applied, CMS may extend the application timeline.

ELIGIBILITY OF BENEFICIARIES TO PARTICIPATE IN THE DEMONSTRATION

To be eligible for the MMHD, Medicare beneficiaries must be covered under Medicare Part A and Part B fee-for-service and must not be enrolled in CMS's hospice, end-stage renal disease, or a Medicare Advantage program. Beneficiaries must have been diagnosed with one or more chronic illnesses that require regular medical monitoring, advising, or treatment, but they must not be long-stay residents of nursing homes. A comprehensive list of qualifying chronic conditions and corresponding International Classification of Diseases (ICD) codes appears in Resource D1: Diagnoses That Make Beneficiaries Eligible for the MMHD at the end of this appendix. Based on these criteria, CMS estimates that approximately 86% of Medicare beneficiaries will be eligible to participate in the demonstration.

Beneficiaries must also agree to participate in a medical home by signing an agreement form that acknowledges the medical home practice and personal physician who will be providing their medical home care. Participation is voluntary, and participating beneficiaries may choose to change practices or disenroll from the demonstration at any time.

CARE MANAGEMENT PAYMENTS TO PARTICIPATING PRACTICES

According to its medical home tier, each medical home will receive a monthly, risk-adjusted fee for each eligible Medicare beneficiary enrolled in the practice, in addition to the traditional fee-for-service payments it receives. The fees for an advanced medical home (Tier 2) will be higher than the fees for a basic medical home (Tier 1) because of the more intense coordination and management services provided by Tier 2 homes.

Care Management and "Shared Savings" Fees During the Demonstration

During the demonstration, CMS will provide risk-adjusted care management payments to the participating medical homes that care for participating beneficiaries. In addition, participating medical homes will be eligible to receive 80% of the net savings to Medicare attributed to the demonstration (over and above the care management payments and traditional encounter-based fee-for-service payments).

Table D.2 shows the amounts of the monthly care management fees that CMS proposes to pay to practices that participate in the MMHD. Payments are higher for Tier 2 practices and for Medicare beneficiaries who are at high risk of using health care services heavily in the next year (i.e., for beneficiaries with HCC values equal to or greater than 1.6). CMS uses the HCC (hierarchical condition category) predictive model and diagnoses from Medicare claims submitted during the previous year to compute each beneficiary's HCC score for the coming year. Care management fees will probably average about $9,700 per month for typical Tier 1 medical homes and about $12,400 per month for typical Tier 2 medical homes. Thus, a typical Tier 2 practice that cared for 240 eligible Medicare beneficiaries could expect to receive care management fees totaling about $149,000 per year during the demonstration.

CMS estimates that approximately 25% of the beneficiaries who enroll in the MMHD will have HCC scores equal to or greater than 1.6. The Office of Management and Budget, must approve this proposal before CMS can implement it.

THE COSTS OF OPERATING A GUIDED CARE MEDICAL HOME, TIER 2

One method for providing Tier 2 medical home services is to adopt Guided Care, use health information technology and deploy a half-time

Table D.2

MONTHLY CARE MANAGEMENT FEES FOR ELIGIBLE MEDICARE BENEFICIARIES ENROLLED IN MEDICAL HOMES

	HCC SCORE < 1.6	HCC SCORE > 1.6	AVERAGE*
Tier 1	$27.12	$80.25	$40.40
Tier 2	$35.48	$100.35	$51.70

Note: Assuming 25% of participating beneficiaries have HCC scores > 1.6.

licensed practical nurse to help provide medical home services. The Guided Care nurse would focus on 50 to 60 of the practice's most complex Medicare beneficiaries, while the licensed practical nurse would facilitate less intense, but complete medical home services to the other participating beneficiaries in the practice. Both would use the medical home features of the practice's health information technology.

As shown in Table D.3, these resources of a Guided Care Tier 2 medical home would cost about $137,400 per year, which is less than the anticipated revenue from CMS's care management payments for a Tier 2 medical home ($149,000 per year). Any "shared savings" from CMS would further expand the revenue available to the practice.

Other types of medical homes would generate different costs and outcomes. A Tier 2 practice in which currently employed physicians, licensed practical nurses, and medical assistants provided all of the required medical home services for all of the practice's eligible Medicare beneficiaries would not incur the costs of a Guided Care nurse or an additional half-time LPN, so it could use the care management fees for health information technology, for office redesign, and for supporting the physicians' and staff members' salaries. Although this model might be successful, its outcomes are unknown. Undoubtedly, a wide range of medical home models will be tested in the MMHD and in other demonstrations of the medical home during the next few years. Careful analysis of the effects of different models on the quality and outcomes of chronic care will provide invaluable information to guide us through the vital transformation of chronic care in America that has just begun.

Table D.3

COSTS OF OPERATING A GUIDED CARE TIER 2 MEDICAL HOME

	SALARY	FRINGE BENEFITS AT 30%	ANNUAL AMOUNT
Licensed practical nurse 0.5 FTE	$21,000	$6,300	$27,300
Guided Care nurse	$71,500[a]	$21,450	$92,950
Electronic health record			$13,000
Guided Care nurse travel: 327 miles/ month at 20 miles/gallon, $3.00/gallon			$587
Equipment (three-year amortization)			
Laptop computer			$600
Cellular telephone			$67
Communication services			
Internet and cellular telephone at $150/month			$1,800
Supplies: patient education booklets			$1,200
Total			**$137,404**

[a]Varies considerably by geographic area and nurse's background.

RESOURCE D1: DIAGNOSES THAT MAKE BENEFICIARIES ELIGIBLE FOR THE MMHD*

Congenital defects

Cardiac and circulatory congenital anomalies: DX 745.0, 745.10, 745.11, 745.12, 745.19, 745.2, 745.3, 745.4, 745.5, 745.60, 745.61, 745.69, 745.7, 745.8, 745.9, 746.00, 746.01, 746.02, 746.09, 746.1, 746.2, 746.3, 746.4, 746.5, 746.6, 746.7, 746.81, 746.82, 746.83, 746.84, 746.85, 746.86, 746.87, 746.89, 746.9, 747.10, 747.11

Digestive congenital anomalies: DX 751.3, 751.60, 751.62, 751.7

Genitourinary congenital anomalies: DX 753.0, 753.12, 753.13, 753.14, 753.16, 753.19, 753.20, 753.29, 753.3

Nervous system congenital anomalies: DX 741.00, 741.01, 741.02, 741.03, 741.90, 741.91, 741.92, 741.93, 742.51

Diseases of the circulatory system

Heart valve disorders: DX 394.0, 394.1, 394.2, 394.9, 395.0, 395.1, 395.2, 395.9, 396.0, 396.1, 396.2, 396.3, 396.8, 396.9, 397.0, 397.1, 397.9, 424.0, 424.1, 424.2, 424.3

Peri-, endo-, and myocarditis, cardiomyopathy (except that caused by tuberculosis or sexually transmitted disease): DX 393, 398.90, 398.99, 423.1, 423.2, 423.8, 423.9, 425.1, 425.4, 425.5, 425.7, 425.8, 425.9, 429.0

Hypertension with complications and secondary hypertension: DX 402.00, 402.10, 402.11, 402.90, 402.91, 403.10, 403.11, 403.90, 403.91, 404.00, 404.10, 404.12, 404.13, 404.90, 405.09, 405.11, 405.19, 405.91, 405.99

Coronary atherosclerosis and other heart disease: DX 412, 413.0, 413.1, 413.9, 414.00, 414.01, 414.8, 414.9

Pulmonary heart disease: DX 416.0, 416.1, 416.8, 416.9, 417.1, 417.8, 417.9

Other and ill-defined heart disease: DX 414.10, 414.11, 414.19, 429.1, 429.2, 429.71, 429.81, 429.82, 429.89, 429.9

Conduction disorders: DX 426.0, 426.10, 426.11, 426.12, 426.13, 426.2, 426.3, 426.4, 426.50, 426.51, 426.52, 426.53, 426.54, 426.6, 426.7, 426.81, 426.89

Cardiac dysrhythmias: DX 427.31, 427.32, 427.81, 427.89, 427.9

Congestive heart failure, nonhypertensive: DX 398.91, 428.0, 428.1, 428.9

Occlusion or stenosis of precerebral arteries: DX 433.00, 433.10, 433.20, 433.30, 433.80, 433.90

Other and ill-defined cerebrovascular disease: DX 437.0, 437.4, 437.8, 437.9

Late effects of cerebrovascular disease: DX 438.0, 438.10, 438.11, 438.12, 438.19, 438.2, 438.20, 438.21, 438.22, 438.30, 438.31, 438.32, 438.4, 438.40, 438.41, 438.42, 438.5, 438.50, 438.51, 438.52, 438.53, 438.81, 438.82, 438.89, 438.9

Peripheral and visceral atherosclerosis: DX 440.0, 440.1, 440.20, 440.21, 440.22, 440.23, 440.29, 440.8, 440.9, 443.9

Aortic, peripheral, and visceral artery aneurysms: DX 441.9

Other circulatory disease: DX 443.1, 443.81, 443.89, 446.0, 446.20, 446.21, 446.3, 446.4, 446.5, 446.7, 447.6, 447.8, 447.9, 448.0, 448.9, 458.1, 459.9

Includes conditions such as esophageal varices without bleeding: DX 456.1, 456.21

Complication of device, implant, or graft: DX 414.02, 414.03, 414.04, 414.05, 440.30, 440.31, 440.32

Diseases of the digestive system

Hepatitis: DX 571.40, 571.41, 571.49

Includes conditions such as chronic vascular insufficiency of intestine (classified by CCS as peripheral and visceral atherosclerosis): DX 557.1, 557.9

Esophageal disorders: DX 530.0, 530.3, 530.5

Other disorders of stomach and duodenum: DX 537.2, 537.6

Regional enteritis and ulcerative colitis: DX 555.0, 555.1, 555.2, 555.9, 556.0, 556.1, 556.2, 556.3, 556.4, 556.5, 556.6, 556.8, 556.9

---

*The codes given are part of the *International Classification of Diseases and Related Health Problems*, 10th revision, published by the World Health Organization.

Liver disease, alcohol-related: DX 571.0, 571.2, 571.3

Other liver diseases: DX 571.5, 571.6, 571.8, 571.9, 572.3, 572.4, 572.8, 573.0, 573.9

Pancreatic disorders (not diabetes): DX 577.1, 577.2, 577.8

Other gastrointestinal disorders: DX 564.81, 579.0, 579.2, 579.3, 579.8, 579.9

Complications of gastric and intestinal surgical procedures or medical care: DX 564.2

Diseases of the urinary and reproductive systems

Nephritis, nephrosis, renal sclerosis: DX 581.0, 581.1, 581.2, 581.3, 581.81, 581.89, 581.9, 582.0, 582.1, 582.2, 582.4, 582.81, 582.89, 582.9, 583.0, 583.1, 583.2, 583.4, 583.6, 583.7, 583.81, 583.89, 583.9, 587

Chronic renal failure: DX 585

Other diseases of kidney and ureters: DX 588.0, 588.1, 588.8, 591, 593.4, 593.71, 593.72, 593.73, 593.9

Other diseases of bladder and urethra: DX 596.4, 596.51, 596.52, 596.53, 596.54, 596.55

Diseases of the musculoskeletal system

Infective arthritis and osteomyelitis (except that caused by tuberculosis or sexually transmitted disease): DX 711.10, 711.19, 730.10, 730.11, 730.12, 730.13, 730.14, 730.15, 730.16, 730.17, 730.18, 730.19, 730.70, 730.71, 730.72, 730.73, 730.74, 730.75, 730.76, 730.77, 730.78, 730.79

Rheumatoid arthritis and related disease: DX 714.0, 714.1, 714.2, 714.30, 714.31, 714.32, 714.33, 714.4, 714.81, 714.89, 720.0

Osteoarthritis: DX 715.00, 715.04, 715.09, 715.10, 715.11, 715.12, 715.13, 715.14, 715.15, 715.16, 715.17, 715.18, 715.20, 715.21, 715.22, 715.23, 715.24, 715.25, 715.26, 715.27, 715.28, 715.30, 715.31, 715.32, 715.33, 715.34, 715.35, 715.36, 715.37, 715.38, 715.80, 715.89, 715.90, 715.91, 715.92, 715.93, 715.94, 715.95, 715.96, 715.97, 715.98

Other nontraumatic joint disorders: DX 713.0, 713.1, 713.2, 713.4, 713.5, 713.7, 718.50, 718.51, 718.52, 718.53, 718.54, 718.55, 718.56, 718.57, 718.58, 718.59, 718.80, 718.81, 718.82, 718.83, 718.84, 718.85, 718.86, 718.87, 718.88, 718.89, 718.90, 718.91, 718.92, 718.93, 718.94, 718.95, 718.97, 718.98, 718.99, 719.90, 719.91, 719.92, 719.93, 719.94, 719.95, 719.96, 719.97, 719.98, 719.99

Spondylosis, intervertebral disc disorders, other back problems: DX 720.1, 720.2, 720.81, 720.89, 721.0, 721.1, 721.2, 721.3, 721.41, 721.42, 721.5, 721.6, 721.8, 721.90, 721.91, 722.0, 722.10, 722.11, 722.2, 722.4, 722.51, 722.52, 722.6, 722.70, 722.71, 722.72, 722.73, 722.80, 722.81, 722.82, 722.83, 723.0, 724.00

Other acquired skeletal deformities: DX 737.10, 737.11, 737.12, 737.19, 737.34, 737.39, 737.40, 737.41, 737.42, 737.43, 738.4

Systemic lupus erythematosis and connective tissue disorders: DX 710.0, 710.1, 710.2, 710.3, 710.4, 710.8, 710.9

Other connective tissue disease: DX 710.5, 725, 726.0, 726.11, 729.0, 729.1

Other bone disease and musculoskeletal deformities: DX 731.0, 731.1, 731.2, 731.8, 733.40, 733.41, 733.42, 733.43, 733.44, 733.49, 733.7, 733.92, 733.99

Diseases of the nervous system

Includes conditions such as Alzheimer's disease (classified by CCS as senility and organic mental disorders): DX 331.0, 331.0, 331.1, 331.2

Parkinson's disease: DX 332.0

Multiple sclerosis: DX 340

Other hereditary and degenerative nervous system conditions: DX 331.3, 331.4, 331.7, 331.89, 331.9, 333.0, 333.2, 333.90, 333.91, 333.99, 334.3, 334.4, 334.8, 334.9, 335.20, 335.22, 335.23, 335.24, 335.29, 335.8, 335.9, 336.0, 336.2, 336.3, 336.9, 337.0, 337.3, 337.9

Paralysis: DX 342.00, 342.01, 342.02, 342.10, 342.11, 342.12, 342.80, 342.81, 342.82, 342.90, 342.91, 342.92, 343.0, 343.1, 343.2, 343.3, 343.4, 343.8, 343.9, 344.00, 344.01, 344.02, 344.03, 344.04, 344.09, 344.1, 344.30, 344.31, 344.32, 344.40, 344.41, 344.42, 344.5, 344.60, 344.81, 344.89, 344.9

Epilepsy, convulsions: DX 45.00, 345.01, 345.10, 345.11, 345.2, 345.40, 345.41, 345.50, 345.51, 345.70, 345.71, 345.80, 345.81, 345.90, 345.91

Headache, including migraine: DX 346.00, 346.01, 346.10, 346.11, 346.20, 346.21, 346.80, 346.81, 346.90, 346.91

Other nervous system disorders: DX 341.0, 341.8, 341.9, 344.61, 347.00, 347.01, 348.0, 350.1, 350.8, 350.9, 352.9, 353.6, 354.4, 354.5, 354.8, 354.9, 355.71, 355.79, 355.8, 355.9, 356.1, 356.2, 356.4, 356.8, 356.9, 357.1, 357.2, 357.3, 357.5, 357.8, 358.0, 358.1, 358.2, 358.8, 358.9, 359.0, 359.1, 359.2, 359.3, 359.5

Diseases of the respiratory system

Chronic obstructive pulmonary disease and bronchiectasis: DX 491.0, 491.1, 491.20, 491.8, 491.9, 492.8, 496

Asthma: DX 493.00, 493.01, 493.10, 493.11, 493.20, 493.21, 493.90, 493.91

Lung disease due to external agents: DX 495.0, 495.1, 495.2, 495.3, 495.4, 495.5, 495.6, 495.7, 495.8, 495.9, 500, 501, 502, 503, 505, 506.4, 508.1

Other lower respiratory disease: DX 515, 516.0, 516.1, 516.3, 516.8, 516.9, 517.2, 517.8, 518.3, 518.89, 519.8, 519.9

Nutritional deficiencies, and metabolic and immunity disorders

Diabetes mellitus without complication: DX 250.00, 250.01, 250.02, 250.03

Diabetes mellitus with complications: DX 250.40, 250.41, 250.42, 250.43, 250.50, 250.51, 250.52, 250.53, 250.60, 250.61, 250.62, 250.63, 250.70, 250.71, 250.72, 250.73, 250.90, 250.91, 250.92, 250.93

Other endocrine disorders: DX 251.1, 251.2, 251.8, 251.9, 252.0, 252.1, 252.9, 253.0, 253.1, 253.2, 253.4, 253.5, 253.6, 253.7, 253.8, 253.9, 255.0, 255.1, 255.3, 255.4, 255.5, 255.8, 255.9, 257.1, 257.2, 258.1, 259.2, 259.3, 259.8, 259.9

Nutritional deficiencies: DX 268.1, 268.2

Gout and other crystal arthropathies: DX 274.10, 274.11, 274.19, 274.81, 274.82, 274.89, 275.0, 275.1, 275.40, 275.49, 275.8, 275.9, 277.1, 277.3, 278.00, 278.01

Cystic fibrosis: DX 277.00, 277.01

Other nutritional, endocrine, and metabolic disorders: DX 273.0, 273.1, 273.2, 273.3, 273.8, 273.9

Mental disorders

Mental retardation: DX 317, 318.0, 318.1, 318.2, 319

Alcohol-related mental disorders: DX 291.0, 291.1, 291.2, 291.3, 291.5, 291.81, 291.89, 291.9, 303.03, 303.90, 303.91, 303.92, 303.93, 305.01, 305.02, 305.03

Substance-related mental disorders: DX 292.0, 304.00, 304.01, 304.02, 304.03, 304.10, 304.11, 304.12, 304.13, 304.20, 304.21, 304.22, 304.23, 304.30, 304.31, 304.32, 304.40, 304.41, 304.42, 304.43, 304.50, 304.51, 304.52, 304.53, 304.60, 304.61, 304.62, 304.63, 304.70, 304.71, 304.72, 304.73, 304.80, 304.81, 304.82, 304.83, 304.90, 304.91, 304.92, 304.93, 305.10, 305.11, 305.12, 305.13, 305.21, 305.23, 305.30, 305.31, 305.32, 305.33, 305.40, 305.41, 305.42, 305.43, 305.50, 305.51, 305.52, 305.53, 305.60, 305.61, 305.62, 305.63, 305.70, 305.71, 305.72, 305.73, 305.80, 305.81, 305.82, 305.83, 305.90, 305.91, 305.92, 305.93

Includes dementias and other persistent mental disorders (classified by CCS as senility and organic mental disorders): DX 290.0, 290.10, 290.11, 290.12, 290.13, 290.20, 290.21, 290.3, 290.40, 290.41, 290.42, 290.43, 290.8, 290.9, 293.1, 293.81, 293.82, 293.83, 293.84, 293.89, 293.9, 294.0, 294.8, 294.9

Anxiety, somatoform, dissociative and personality disorders: DX 300.00, 300.01, 300.02, 300.09, 300.23, 300.5, 300.7, 300.81, 300.82, 307.40, 307.42, 307.44, 307.80, 307.81, 307.89, 307.9, 309.81

Other mental conditions: DX 300.89, 300.9, 306.0, 306.1, 306.2, 306.3, 306.4, 306.50, 309.1, 311

Cancers

Cancer of head and neck: DX 140.0, 140.1, 140.3, 140.4, 140.5, 140.6, 140.8, 140.9, 141.0, 141.1, 141.2, 141.3, 141.4, 141.5, 141.6, 141.8, 141.9, 142.0, 142.1, 142.2, 142.8, 142.9, 143.0, 143.1, 143.8, 143.9, 144.0, 144.1, 144.8, 144.9, 145.0, 145.1, 145.2, 145.3, 145.4, 145.5, 145.6, 145.8, 145.9, 146.0, 146.1, 146.2, 146.3, 146.4, 146.5, 146.6, 146.7, 146.8, 146.9, 147.0, 147.1, 147.2, 147.3, 147.8, 147.9, 148.0, 148.1, 148.2, 148.3, 148.8, 148.9, 149.0, 149.1, 149.8, 149.9, 160.0, 160.1, 160.2, 160.3, 160.4, 160.5, 160.8, 160.9, 161.0, 161.1, 161.2, 161.3, 161.8, 161.9, 195

Cancer of esophagus: DX 150.0, 150.1, 150.2, 150.3, 150.4, 150.5, 150.8, 150.9

Cancer of stomach: DX 151.0, 151.1, 151.2, 151.3, 151.4, 151.5, 151.6, 151.8, 151.9

Cancer of colon: DX 153.0, 153.1, 153.2, 153.3, 153.4, 153.5, 153.6, 153.7, 153.8, 153.9, 159.0

Cancer of rectum and anus: DX 154.0, 154.1, 154.2, 154.3, 154.8

Cancer of liver and intrahepatic bile duct: DX 155.0, 155.1, 155.2

Cancer of pancreas: DX 157.0, 157.1, 157.2, 157.3, 157.4, 157.8, 157.9

Cancer of other gastrointestinal (GI) organs, peritoneum: DX 152.0, 152.1, 152.2, 152.3, 152.8, 152.9, 156.0, 156.1, 156.2, 156.8, 156.9, 158.0, 158.8, 158.9, 159.1, 159.8, 159.9

Cancer of bronchus, lung: DX 162.2, 162.3, 162.4, 162.5, 162.8, 162.9

Cancer, other respiratory and intrathoracic: DX 162.0, 162.3, 162.4, 162.5, 162.8, 162.9, 163.0, 163.1, 163.8, 163.9, 164.0, 164.1, 164.2, 164.3, 164.8, 164.9, 165.0, 165.8, 165.9

Cancer of bone and connective tissue: DX 170.0, 170.1, 170.2, 170.3, 170.4, 170.5, 170.6, 170.7, 170.8, 170.9, 171.0, 171.2, 171.3, 171.4, 171.5, 171.6, 171.7, 171.8, 171.9

Melanomas of skin: DX 172.0, 172.1, 172.2, 172.3, 172.4, 172.5, 172.6, 172.7, 172.8, 172.9

Cancer of breast: DX 174.0, 174.1, 174.2, 174.3, 174.4, 174.5, 174.6, 174.8, 174.9, 175.0, 175.9

Cancer of uterus: DX 179, 182.0, 182.1, 182.8

Cancer of cervix: DX 180.0, 180.1, 180.8, 180.9

Cancer of ovary: DX 183

Cancer of other female genital organs: DX 181, 183.2, 183.3, 183.4, 183.5, 183.8, 183.9, 184.0, 184.1, 184.2, 184.3, 184.4, 184.8, 184.9

Cancer of prostate: DX 185

Cancer of testis: DX 186.0, 186.9

Cancer of other male genital organs: DX 187.1, 187.2, 187.3, 187.4, 187.5, 187.6, 187.7, 187.8, 187.9

Cancer of bladder: DX 188, 188.0, 188.1, 188.2, 188.3, 188.4, 188.5, 188.6, 188.7, 188.8, 188.9

Cancer of kidney and renal pelvis: DX 189.0, 189.1

Cancer of other urinary organs: DX 189.2, 189.3, 189.4, 189.8, 189.9

Cancer of brain and nervous system: DX 191.0, 191.1, 191.1, 191.2, 191.3, 191.4, 191.5, 191.6, 191.7, 191.8, 191.9, 192.0, 192.1, 192.2, 192.3, 192.8, 192.9

Cancer of thyroid: DX 193

Hodgkin's disease: DX 201.00, 201.01, 201.02, 201.03, 201.04, 201.05, 201.06, 201.07, 201.08, 201.10, 201.11, 201.12, 201.13, 201.14, 201.15, 201.16, 201.17, 201.18, 201.20, 201.21, 201.22, 201.23, 201.24, 201.25, 201.26, 201.27, 201.28, 201.40, 201.41, 201.42, 201.43, 201.44, 201.45, 201.46, 201.47, 201.48, 201.50, 201.51, 201.52, 201.53, 201.54, 201.55, 201.56, 201.57, 201.58, 201.60, 201.61, 201.62, 201.63, 201.64, 201.65, 201.66, 201.67, 201.68, 201.70, 201.71, 201.72, 201.73, 201.74, 201.75, 201.76, 201.77, 201.78, 201.90, 201.91, 201.92, 201.93, 201.94, 201.95, 201.96, 201.97, 201.98

Non-Hodgkin's lymphoma: DX 200.00, 200.01, 200.02, 200.03, 200.04, 200.05, 200.06, 200.07, 200.08, 200.10, 200.11, 200.12, 200.13, 200.14, 200.15, 200.16, 200.17, 200.18, 200.80, 200.81, 200.82, 200.83, 200.84, 200.85, 200.86, 200.87, 200.88, 202.00, 202.01, 202.02, 202.03, 202.04, 202.05, 202.06, 202.07, 202.08, 202.10, 202.11, 202.12, 202.13, 202.14, 202.15, 202.16, 202.17, 202.18, 202.20, 202.21, 202.22, 202.23, 202.24, 202.25, 202.26, 202.27, 202.28, 202.80, 202.81, 202.82, 202.83, 202.84, 202.85, 202.86, 202.87, 202.88, 202.90, 202.91, 202.92, 202.93, 202.94, 202.95, 202.96, 202.97, 202.98

Leukemias: DX 202.40, 202.41, 202.42, 202.43, 202.44, 202.45, 202.46, 202.47, 202.48, 203.10, 203.11, 204.00, 204.01, 204.10, 204.11, 204.20, 204.21, 204.80, 204.81, 204.90, 204.91, 205.00, 205.01, 205.10, 205.11, 205.20, 205.21, 205.30, 205.31, 205.80, 205.81, 205.90, 205.91, 206.00, 206.01, 206.10, 206.11, 206.20, 206.21, 206.80, 206.81, 206.90, 206.91, 207.00, 207.01, 207.10, 207.11, 207.20, 207.21, 207.80, 207.81, 208.00, 208.01, 208.10, 208.11, 208.20, 208.21, 208.80, 208.81, 208.90, 208.91

Multiple myeloma: DX 203.00, 203.01, 203.80, 203.81

Cancer, other and unspecified primary: DX 176.0, 176.1, 176.2, 176.3, 176.4, 176.5, 176.8, 176.9, 194.0, 194.1, 194.3, 194.4, 194.5, 194.6, 194.8, 194.9, 195.1, 195.2, 195.3, 195.4, 195.5, 195.8, 202.30, 202.31, 202.32, 202.33, 202.34, 202.35, 202.36, 202.37, 202.38

Secondary malignancies: DX 196.0, 196.1, 196.1, 196.2, 196.3, 196.5, 196.6, 196.8, 196.9, 197.0, 197.1, 197.2, 197.3, 197.4, 197.5, 197.6, 197.7, 197.8, 198.0, 198.1, 198.2, 198.3, 198.4, 198.5, 198.6, 198.7, 198.81, 198.82, 198.89

Malignant neoplasm without specification of site: DX 199.0, 199.1

Neoplasms of unspecified nature or uncertain behavior: DX 236.90, 237.70, 237.71, 237.72, 238.4, 238.5, 238.6, 238.7

Injury and poisoning

Fracture of neck of femur (hip): DX 905.3

Spinal cord injury: DX 907.2

Crushing injury or internal injury: DX 906.4, 908.0, 908.1, 908.2, 908.3, 908.4

Complications of surgical procedures or medical care: DX 909.3, 997.62

Burns: DX 906.5

Blood-related diseases

Deficiency and other anemia: DX 284.8, 284.9

Sickle cell anemia: DX 282.60, 282.61, 282.63, 282.69

Coagulation and hemorrhagic disorders: DX 286.0, 286.1, 286.2, 286.3, 286.4, 287.1, 287.3

Other hematologic conditions: DX 289.4, 289.6, 289.8, 289.9

Infectious and parasitic diseases

HIV infection: DX 042.0, 042.1, 042.2, 042.9, 043, 043.0, 043.1, 043.2, 043.3, 043.9, 044, 044.0, 044.9

Hepatitis: DX 070.54

Non-organ-specific symptoms

Senility and organic mental disorders: DX 797

Malaise and fatigue: DX 780.71

Supplementary classification

HIV infection: DX V08

Other liver diseases: DX V42.7

Other nervous system disorders: DX V45.2

Heart valve disorders: DX V42.2, V43.3

Coronary atherosclerosis and other heart disease: DX V45.81

Conduction disorders: DX V45.00, V45.01, V45.02, V45.09

Other circulatory disease: DX V42.1, V43.2

Other lower respiratory disease: DX V42.6

Chronic renal failure: DX V45.1

Other connective tissue disease: DX V43.60, V43.61, V43.62, V43.63, V43.64, V43.65, V43.66, V43.69, V43.7

Rehabilitation care, fitting of prostheses, and adjustment of devices: DX V52.0, V52.1, V52.4

Conditions not to be used for assessing eligibility

Cancer of the head and neck: DX 140, 141, 142, 143, 144, 145, 146, 147, 148, 149, 160, 161

Cancer of esophagus: DX 150

Cancer of stomach: DX 151

Cancer of other GI organs, peritoneum: DX 152, 156, 158

Cancer of colon: DX 153, 159

Cancer of rectum and anus: DX 154

Cancer of liver and intrahepatic bile duct: DX 155

Cancer of pancreas: DX 157

Cancer, other respiratory and intrathoracic: DX 162, 163, 165

Cancer, other and unspecified primary: DX 164, 176, 190, 190.0, 190.1, 190.2, 190.3, 190.4, 190.5, 190.6, 190.7, 190.8, 190.9, 194, 195, 202.3, 202.5, 202.50, 202.51, 202.52, 202.53, 202.54, 202.55, 202.56, 202.57, 202.58, 202.6, 202.60, 202.61, 202.62, 202.63, 202.64, 202.65, 202.66, 202.67, 202.68

Cancer of bone and connective tissue: DX 170, 171

Melanomas of the skin: DX 172

Other non-epithelial cancer of skin: DX 173, 173.0, 173.1, 173.2, 173.3, 173.4, 173.5, 173.6, 173.7, 173.8, 173.9

Cancer of breast: DX 174, 175

Cancer of cervix: DX 180

Cancer of uterus: DX 182

Cancer of ovary: DX 183

Cancer of other female genital organs: DX 184

Cancer of testis: DX 186

Cancer of other male genital organs: DX 187

Cancer of kidney and renal pelvis: DX 189

Cancer of brain and nervous system: DX 191, 192

Secondary malignancies: DX 196, 197, 198, 198.8

Malignant neoplasm without specification of site: DX 199

Non-Hodgkin's lymphoma: DX 200, 200.0, 200.1, 200.2, 200.20, 200.21, 200.22, 200.23, 200.24, 200.25, 200.26, 200.27, 200.28, 200.8, 202, 202.0, 202.1, 202.2, 202.8, 202.9

Hodgkin's disease: DX 201, 201.0, 201.1, 201.2, 201.4, 201.5, 201.6, 201.7, 201.9

Multiple myeloma: DX 203, 203.0, 203.8

Leukemias: DX 203.1, 204, 204.0, 204.1, 204.2, 204.8, 204.9, 205, 205.0, 205.1, 205.2, 205.3, 205.8, 205.9, 206, 206.0, 206.1, 206.2, 206.8, 206.9, 207, 207.0, 207.1, 207.2, 207.8, 208, 208.0, 208.1, 208.2, 208.8, 208.9

Neoplasms of unspecified nature or uncertain behavior: DX 237.7

Tuberculosis: DX 137, 137.0, 137.1, 137.2, 137.3, 137.4

Bacterial infection, unspecified site: DX 030, 030.0, 030.1, 030.2, 030.3, 030.8, 030.9, 040.1

Viral infection: DX 053.12, 053.13, 079.5, 079.50, 079.51, 079.52, 079.59

Other infections, including parasitic: DX 086, 086.0, 086.2, 102.5, 102.6, 125.0, 125.1, 125.5, 125.6, 135, 139.8

Sexually transmitted infections (not HIV or hepatitis): DX 090.5, 090.7, 091.50, 093.1, 093.22, 093.24, 093.9, 094.0, 094.1, 094.3, 094.82, 094.83, 094.86, 095.0, 095.0, 095.1, 095.2, 095.3, 095.4, 095.5, 095.6, 095.7, 095.8, 095.9, 099.3

Human immunodeficiency virus (HIV) Infection: DX 042, 079.53, 279.10, 279.10, 279.19, 279.19, 795.8

Hepatitis: DX 070.30

Immunizations and screening for infectious disease: DX V02.6, V02.60, V02.61, V02.62, V02.69

Maintenance chemotherapy, radiotherapy: DX V58.0, V58.1, V67.1, V67.2

Thyroid disorders: DX 240, 240.0, 240.9, 241, 241.0, 241.1, 241.9, 242, 242.0, 242.00, 242.01, 242.1, 242.10, 242.2, 242.20, 242.3, 242.30, 242.4, 242.40, 242.41, 242.8, 242.80, 242.81, 242.9, 242.90, 242.91, 243, 244, 244.0, 244.1, 244.2, 244.3, 244.8, 244.9, 245, 245.2, 245.3, 245.8, 246, 246.0, 246.1, 246.8, 246.9

Diabetes mellitus without complication: DX 250, 250.0

Diabetes mellitus with complication: DX 250.4, 250.5, 250.6, 250.7, 250.8, 250.9

Other endocrine disorders: DX 251, 251.4, 251.5, 252, 253, 253.3, 255, 255.2, 256.4, 258, 258.0, 258.8, 258.9, 259

Nutritional deficiencies: DX 268

Other nutritional, endocrine, and metabolic disorders: DX 270, 270.0, 270.1, 270.2, 270.3, 270.4, 270.5, 270.6, 270.7, 270.8, 270.9, 271, 271.0, 271.03, 271.1, 271.2, 271.3, 271.4, 271.8, 271.9, 272.5, 272.6, 272.7, 272.8, 272.9, 273, 275, 275.3, 275.4, 277.2, 277.5, 277.6, 277.8, 277.9, 278, 278.0, 278.4

Disorders of lipid metabolism: DX 272, 272.0, 272.00, 272.1, 272.2, 272.3, 272.4

Gout and other crystal arthropathies: DX 274.1

Cystic fibrosis: DX 277.0

Immunity disorders: DX 279, 279.0, 279.00, 279.01, 279.02, 279.03, 279.04, 279.05, 279.06, 279.09, 279.1, 279.11, 279.12, 279.13, 279.2, 279.3, 279.4, 279.8, 279.9

Conditions not to be used for assessing eligibility *(continued)*

Deficiency and other anemia: DX 281, 281.0, 281.1, 281.3, 282, 282.0, 282.1, 282.2, 282.3, 282.4, 282.7, 282.8, 282.9, 284, 284.0, 288.1, 288.2

Sickle cell anemia: DX 282.6

Senility and organic mental disorders: DX 290, 290.1, 290.2, 290.4, 293, 293.8, 294, 294.1, 310, 331

Alcohol-related mental disorders: DX 291, 291.12, 291.8, 303, 303.0, 303.00, 303.01, 303.02, 303.9

Substance-related mental disorders: DX 292, 304, 304.0, 304.1, 304.2, 304.3, 304.4, 304.5, 304.6, 304.7, 304.8, 304.9, 305.0, 305.2, 305.3, 305.4, 305.5, 305.6, 305.7, 305.8, 305.9

Schizophrenia and related disorders: DX 295, 295.0, 295.00, 295.01, 295.02, 295.03, 295.04, 295.05, 295.1, 295.10, 295.11, 295.12, 295.13, 295.14, 295.15, 295.2, 295.20, 295.21, 295.22, 295.23, 295.24, 295.25, 295.3, 295.30, 295.31, 295.32, 295.33, 295.34, 295.35, 295.4, 295.40, 295.41, 295.42, 295.43, 295.44, 295.45, 295.5, 295.50, 295.51, 295.52, 295.53, 295.54, 295.55, 295.6, 295.60, 295.61, 295.62, 295.63, 295.64, 295.65, 295.7, 295.70, 295.71, 295.72, 295.73, 295.74, 295.75, 295.8, 295.80, 295.81, 295.82, 295.83, 295.84, 295.85, 295.9, 295.90, 295.91, 295.92, 295.93, 295.94, 295.95, 299, 299.0, 299.00, 299.01, 299.1, 299.10, 299.11, 299.8, 299.80, 299.81, 299.9, 299.90, 299.91

Affective disorders: DX 296, 296.0, 296.00, 296.01, 296.02, 296.03, 296.04, 296.05, 296.06, 296.1, 296.10, 296.11, 296.12, 296.13, 296.14, 296.15, 296.16, 296.2, 296.20, 296.21, 296.22, 296.23, 296.24, 296.25, 296.26, 296.3, 296.30, 296.31, 296.32, 296.33, 296.34, 296.35, 296.36, 296.4, 296.40, 296.41, 296.42, 296.43, 296.44, 296.45, 296.46, 296.5, 296.50, 296.51, 296.52, 296.53, 296.54, 296.55, 296.56, 296.6, 296.60, 296.61, 296.62, 296.63, 296.64, 296.65, 296.66, 296.7, 296.8, 296.80, 296.81, 296.82, 296.89, 296.9, 296.90, 296.99, 298, 298.0, 301.11, 301.13

Other psychoses: DX 297, 297.0, 297.1, 297.2, 297.3, 297.8, 297.9, 298.1, 298.2, 298.3, 298.4, 298.8, 298.9

Anxiety, somatoform, dissociative and personality disorders: DX 300, 300.0, 300.13, 300.14, 300.15, 300.16, 300.19, 300.2, 300.20, 300.21, 300.22, 300.29, 300.3, 300.4, 300.6, 300.8, 301, 301.0, 301.1, 301.10, 301.12, 301.2, 301.20, 301.21, 301.22, 301.3, 301.4, 301.5, 301.50, 301.51, 301.59, 301.6, 301.7, 301.8, 301.81, 301.82, 301.83, 301.84, 301.89, 301.9, 307.8, 312.3, 312.30, 312.31, 312.32, 312.33, 312.34, 312.35, 312.39, 312.90

Other mental conditions: DX 302.1, 302.2, 302.3, 302.4, 302.5, 302.50, 302.51, 302.52, 302.53, 302.6, 302.8, 302.81, 302.82, 302.83, 302.84, 302.85, 302.89, 302.9, 306, 306.5, 306.51, 306.52, 306.53, 306.59, 306.6, 306.7, 306.8, 306.9, 307, 307.0, 307.1, 307.2, 307.20, 307.22, 307.23, 307.3, 307.5, 307.50, 307.51, 307.52, 307.53, 307.54, 307.59, 307.6, 307.7, 313.1, 313.22, 313.23, 313.3, 313.3, 313.81, 313.83, 313.89, 313.9, 315, 315.0, 315.00, 315.01, 315.02, 315.09, 315.1, 315.2, 315.3, 315.31, 315.32, 315.39, 315.4, 315.5, 315.8, 315.9, 316

Preadult disorders: DX 309.21, 312, 312.0, 312.00, 312.01, 312.02, 312.03, 312.1, 312.10, 312.11, 312.12, 312.13, 312.2, 312.20, 312.21, 312.22, 312.23, 312.4, 312.8, 312.81, 312.82, 312.89, 312.9, 313, 313.0, 313.2, 313.21, 314, 314.0, 314.00, 314.01, 314.1, 314.2, 314.8, 314.9

Mental retardation: DX 318

Meningitis (except that caused by tuberculosis or sexually transmitted disease): DX 322.2

Encephalitis (except that caused by tuberculosis or sexually transmitted disease): DX 046.2, 139, 139.0

Other central nervous system (CNS) infection and poliomyelitis: DX 046, 046.0, 046.1, 046.3, 046.8, 046.9, 138, 326

Other hereditary and degenerative nervous system conditions: DX 330, 330.0, 330.1, 330.2, 330.3, 330.8, 330.9, 331.8, 333, 333.4, 333.6, 333.7, 333.9, 333.93, 334, 334.0, 334.1, 334.2, 335, 335.0, 335.1, 335.10, 335.11, 335.19, 335.2, 335.21, 336, 337

Parkinson's disease: DX 332

Other nervous system disorders: DX 341, 341.1, 347.0, 347.1, 350, 352, 354, 355, 355.1, 355.7, 356, 356.0, 356.3, 358, 359

Paralysis: DX 342, 342.0, 342.1, 342.9, 343, 344.0, 344.3, 344.4, 344.6, 344.8

Epilepsy, convulsions: DX 345, 345.0, 345.1, 345.4, 345.5, 345.6, 345.60, 345.61, 345.7, 345.8, 345.9

Headache, including migraine: DX 346, 346.0, 346.1, 346.2, 346.8, 346.9

Cataract: DX 366, 366.0, 366.00, 366.01, 366.02, 366.03, 366.04, 366.09, 366.1, 366.10, 366.11, 366.12, 366.13, 366.14, 366.15, 366.16, 366.17, 366.19, 366.3, 366.30, 366.31, 366.32, 366.33, 366.34, 366.4, 366.41, 366.42, 366.43, 366.44, 366.45, 366.46, 366.5, 366.50, 366.51, 366.52, 366.53, 366.8, 366.9, V43, V43.1

Retinal detachments, defects, vascular occlusion, and retinopathy: DX 361.06, 361.07, 361.1, 361.10, 361.11, 361.12, 361.13, 361.14, 361.19, 361.2, 361.3, 361.30, 361.31, 361.33, 362, 362.0, 362.01, 362.02, 362.1, 362.10, 362.11, 362.12, 362.15, 362.16, 362.17, 362.18, 362.2, 362.21, 362.29, 362.3, 362.30, 362.31, 362.32, 362.33, 362.35, 362.36, 362.4, 362.40, 362.41, 362.42, 362.43, 362.5, 362.50, 362.51, 362.52, 362.53, 362.54, 362.56, 362.57, 362.6, 362.60, 362.61, 362.62, 362.63, 362.64, 362.65, 362.66, 362.7, 362.70, 362.71, 362.72, 362.73, 362.74, 362.75, 362.76, 362.77

Glaucoma: DX 365, 365.0, 365.00, 365.01, 365.02, 365.04, 365.1, 365.10, 365.11, 365.12, 365.13, 365.14, 365.15, 365.2, 365.20, 365.21, 365.23, 365.24, 365.31, 365.4, 365.41, 365.42, 365.43, 365.44, 365.5, 365.51, 365.52, 365.59, 365.6, 365.60, 365.61, 365.62, 365.63, 365.64, 365.8, 365.81, 365.82, 365.89, 365.9

Inflammation, infection of eye (except that caused by tuberculosis or sexually transmitted disease): DX 054.4, 054.42, 054.43, 054.44, 054.49, 055.71, 115.02, 139.1, 360.03, 360.12, 363, 363.0, 363.00, 363.01, 363.03, 363.04, 363.05, 363.06, 363.07, 363.08, 363.1, 363.10, 363.11, 363.12, 363.13, 363.14, 363.15, 363.2, 363.20, 363.21, 363.22, 364, 364.1, 364.10, 364.11, 364.2, 364.21, 364.24, 364.3, 370.23, 370.3, 370.31, 370.32, 370.33, 370.35, 370.5, 370.50, 370.52, 370.54, 370.59, 370.8, 372.1, 372.10, 372.11, 372.12, 372.13, 372.14, 372.15, 372.2, 372.20, 372.21, 372.22, 372.3, 372.31, 372.39, 373, 373.00, 373.01, 375.0, 375.02, 375.41, 375.42, 376.1, 376.10, 376.11, 376.12, 376.13, 377.33, 379.0, 379.00, 379.04, 379.05, 379.07

Mycoses: DX 117.0, 117.4

Other eye disorders: DX 360.2, 360.20, 360.21, 360.23, 360.24, 360.29, 360.4, 360.40, 360.41, 360.42, 360.5, 360.50, 360.51, 360.52, 360.53, 360.54, 360.55, 360.59, 363.4, 363.40, 363.41, 363.42, 360.10, 363.5, 363.50, 363.51, 363.52, 363.53, 363.54, 363.55, 363.56, 363.57, 364.5, 364.51, 364.53, 364.54, 364.55, 364.56, 364.57, 364.59, 364.6, 364.60, 364.61, 364.62, 364.63, 364.64, 364.76, 364.77, 364.8, 364.9, 370.01, 370.02, 370.03, 370.04, 370.05, 370.07, 371, 371.0, 371.00, 371.03, 371.04, 371.05, 371.23, 371.4, 371.40, 371.42, 371.43, 371.44, 371.45, 371.46, 371.48, 371.49, 371.5, 371.50, 371.51, 371.52, 371.53, 371.54, 371.55, 371.56, 371.57, 371.58, 371.6, 371.60, 371.61, 371.7, 371.70, 371.71, 371.73, 371.81, 372.5, 372.50, 372.51, 372.52, 372.53, 372.54, 372.55, 372.56, 372.6, 372.61, 372.62, 372.63, 372.64, 372.8, 372.9, 374.0, 374.05, 374.1, 374.10, 374.11, 374.12, 374.13, 374.14, 374.2, 374.21, 374.22, 374.23, 374.43, 374.46, 374.50, 375.1, 375.15, 376.2, 376.21, 376.22, 377.11, 377.12, 377.13, 377.16, 377.2, 377.21, 377.22, 377.23, 377.41, 377.5, 377.51, 377.52, 377.53, 377.54, 377.6, 377.61, 377.62, 377.63, 377.7, 377.71, 377.72, 377.73, 377.75, 377.9, 378, 378.0, 378.00, 378.01, 378.02, 378.03, 378.04, 378.05, 378.06, 378.07, 378.08, 378.1, 378.10, 378.11, 378.12, 378.13, 378.14, 378.15, 378.16, 378.17, 378.18, 378.2, 378.20, 378.21, 378.22, 378.23, 378.24, 378.3, 378.30, 378.31, 378.32, 378.33, 378.34, 378.35, 378.4, 378.40, 378.41, 378.42, 378.43, 378.44, 378.45, 378.7, 378.71, 378.72, 378.73, 378.8, 378.82, 378.83, 378.84, 378.85, 379.1, 379.11, 379.12, 379.13, 379.14, 379.15, 379.16, 379.19, 379.2, 379.23, 379.24, 379.25, 379.26, 379.29, 379.3, 379.31, 379.32, 379.33, 379.34, 379.39, 379.53, 379.54, 379.55, V52.2

Blindness and vision defects: DX 367, 367.0, 367.1, 367.2, 367.20, 367.21, 367.22, 367.3, 367.31, 367.32, 367.4, 367.51, 367.53, 367.89, 367.9, 368, 368.0, 368.00, 368.01, 368.02, 368.03, 368.3, 368.30, 368.31, 368.32, 368.6, 369, 369.0, 369.00, 369.01, 369.02, 369.03, 369.04, 369.05, 369.06, 369.07, 369.08, 369.1, 369.10, 369.11, 369.12, 369.13, 369.14, 369.15, 369.16, 369.17, 369.18, 369.2, 369.20, 369.21, 369.22, 369.23, 369.24, 369.25, 369.3, 369.4, 369.6, 369.60, 369.61, 369.62, 369.63, 369.64, 369.65, 369.66, 369.67, 369.68, 369.69, 369.7, 369.70, 369.71, 369.72, 369.73, 369.74, 369.75, 369.76, 369.8, 369.9

Other ear and sense organ disorders: DX 380.02, 380.16, 380.5, 380.50, 380.53, 385.3, 385.30, 385.31, 385.32, 385.33, 385.35, 385.8, 385.82, 385.83, 385.89, 385.9, 388.0, 388.00, 388.01, 388.5, 389, 389.1, 389.10, 389.11, 389.12, 389.14, 389.18, 389.7, 389.9

Otitis media and related conditions: DX 381.19, 381.5, 381.52, 381.6, 381.61, 381.62, 381.81, 383.1, 383.3, 383.30, 383.32, 383.33, 383.89, 384.8, 384.81, 384.82, 385, 385.0, 385.00, 385.01, 385.02, 385.03, 385.09, 385.1, 385.10, 385.11, 385.12, 385.13, 385.19, 385.2, 385.21, 385.22, 385.23, 385.24, 387, 387.0, 387.1, 387.2, 387.8, 387.9

Conditions associated with dizziness or vertigo: DX 386, 386.0, 386.00, 386.01, 386.02, 386.03, 386.10, 386.12, 386.58, 386.9

Heart valve disorders: DX 394, 395, 396, 397, 424

Peri-, endo-, and myocarditis, cardiomyopathy (except that caused by tuberculosis or sexually transmitted disease): DX 398, 398.9, 423, 425, 425.0, 425.2, 425.3, 429

Essential hypertension: DX 401, 401.1, 401.9

Hypertension with complications and secondary hypertension: DX 402, 402.0, 402.1, 402.9, 403, 403.1, 403.9, 404, 404.0, 404.1, 404.9, 405, 405.1, 405.9

Conditions not to be used for assessing eligibility *(continued)*

Coronary atherosclerosis and other heart disease: DX 413, 414, 414.0

Other and ill-defined heart disease: DX 414.1, 429.8, 437, 437.5

Pulmonary heart disease: DX 416, 417

Conduction disorders: DX 426, 426.1, 426.5, 426.8, V45.0

Cardiac dysrhythmias: DX 427, 427.3, 427.8

Congestive heart failure, nonhypertensive: DX 428

Occlusion or stenosis of precerebral arteries: DX 433, 433.0, 433.1, 433.2, 433.3, 433.8, 433.9

Late effects of cerebrovascular disease: DX 438, 438.1, 438.3, 438.8

Peripheral and visceral atherosclerosis: DX 440, 440.2, 557

Aortic, peripheral, and visceral artery aneurysms: DX 441

Other circulatory disease: DX 443, 443.8, 446, 447, 448

Esophageal disorders: DX 456.2, 530

Other diseases of veins and lymphatics: DX 459, 459.1, 459.8, 459.81

Pneumonia (except that caused by tuberculosis or sexually transmitted disease): DX 517, 517.1

Pleurisy, pneumothorax, pulmonary collapse: DX 518.1, 518.2

Respiratory failure, insufficiency, arrest (adult): DX 518.8, 518.81, 518.83, 518.84, V46.1

Other upper respiratory disease: DX 471.1, 476, 476.0, 476.1, 478.3, 478.30, 478.31, 478.32, 478.33, 478.34, V44, V44.0

Chronic obstructive pulmonary disease and bronchiectasis: DX 491, 491.2, 492, 494

Asthma: DX 493, 493.0, 493.1, 493.2, 493.9

Lung disease due to external agents: DX 495, 508

Other lower respiratory disease: DX 516, 516.2

Disorders of teeth and jaw: DX 524.8

Diseases of mouth, excluding dental: DX 527.7

Gastritis and duodenitis: DX 535.1

Regional enteritis and ulcerative colitis: DX 555, 556

Other gastrointestinal disorders: DX 564.1, 564.5, 564.8, 564.89, 564.9, 579, 579.1

Liver disease, alcohol-related: DX 571

Hepatitis: DX 571.4

Other liver diseases: DX 572

Nephritis, nephrosis, renal sclerosis: DX 581, 581.8, 582, 582.8, 583, 583.8

Acute and unspecified renal failure: DX 586

Other diseases of kidney and ureters: DX 588, 596.5

Urinary tract infections: DX 590.0, 590.00, 595.1

Hyperplasia of prostate: DX 600

Inflammatory conditions of male genital organs: DX 601.1

Other male genital disorders: DX 607.8, 607.84, 607.89

Nonmalignant breast conditions : DX 610, 610.1, 610.2, 610.3, 610.4, 610.8, 610.9

Endometriosis : DX 617, 617.0, 617.1, 617.2, 617.3, 617.4, 617.5, 617.6, 617.8, 617.9

Menstrual disorders: DX 625.3

Other female genital disorders: DX 625.4, 625.6, 625.8

Other complications of pregnancy: DX 648.1, 648.10, 648.11, 648.12, 648.13, 648.14, 648.40, 648.5, 648.50, 648.51, 648.52, 648.53, 648.54, 648.7, 648.70, 648.71, 648.72, 648.73, 648.74

Hypertension complicating pregnancy, childbirth, and the puerperium: DX 642.0, 642.00, 642.01, 642.02, 642.03, 642.04, 642.1, 642.10, 642.11, 642.12, 642.13, 642.14, 642.2, 642.20, 642.21, 642.22, 642.23, 642.24

Diabetes or abnormal glucose tolerance complicating pregnancy, childbirth, or the puerperium: DX 648.0, 648.00, 648.01, 648.02, 648.04

Other inflammatory condition of skin: DX 694.61, 696.0

Chronic ulcer of skin: DX 707, 707.1, 707.9

Other skin disorders: DX 704.01

Systemic lupus erythematosus and connective tissue disorders: DX 710

Infective arthritis and osteomyelitis (except that caused by tuberculosis or sexually transmitted disease): DX 711.1, 730.1, 730.7

Other nontraumatic joint disorders: DX 713

Rheumatoid arthritis and related disease: DX 714, 714.3, 714.8, 720

Osteoarthritis: DX 715, 715.0, 715.06, 715.1, 715.2, 715.3, 715.8, 715.86, 715.87, 715.9, 715.99

Other nontraumatic joint disorders: DX 716.01, 716.02, 716.03, 716.04, 716.05, 718.5, 718.8, 718.9, 719.2, 719.20, 719.21, 719.22, 719.23, 719.24, 719.25, 719.26, 719.27, 719.28, 719.29, 719.9

Spondylosis, intervertebral disc disorders, other back problems: DX 720.8, 721, 721.4, 721.9, 722, 722.1, 722.5, 722.7, 722.8, 724.0

Other connective tissue disease: DX 726.61, 726.62, 726.63, 728.1, 728.10, 728.11, 728.12, 728.19, 728.3, 729, 729.91, V43.6

Other bone disease and musculoskeletal deformities: DX 731, 732, 732.0, 732.1, 732.2, 732.3, 732.4, 732.5, 732.6, 732.7, 732.8, 733.4, 733.5

Osteoporosis: DX 733.0, 733.00, 733.01, 733.02, 733.03, 733.09

Acquired foot deformities: DX 735.2, 735.3, 735.4, 735.5, 735.8, 735.9

Other acquired deformities: DX 736.1, 737.1, 737.4

Nervous system congenital anomalies: DX 740.1, 740.2, 741, 741.0, 741.9, 742, 742.0, 742.1, 742.2, 742.3, 742.4, 742.5, 742.53, 742.9

Other congenital anomalies: DX 743.0, 743.00, 743.03, 743.06, 743.1, 743.10, 743.12, 743.2, 743.20, 743.21, 743.22, 743.32, 743.33, 743.34, 743.35, 743.36, 743.37, 743.39, 743.4, 743.41, 743.42, 743.43, 743.44, 743.45, 743.46, 743.47, 743.48, 743.49, 743.5, 743.51, 743.52, 743.53, 743.54, 743.55, 743.56, 743.57, 743.58, 743.59, 743.6, 743.61, 743.62, 743.63, 743.64, 743.65, 743.66, 743.69, 743.8, 743.9, 748.4, 748.5, 748.6, 748.60, 748.61, 748.69, 754.3, 754.30, 754.31, 754.32, 754.33, 754.35, 756, 756.1, 756.11, 756.12, 756.13, 756.14, 756.15, 756.16, 756.17, 756.4, 756.5, 756.50, 756.51, 756.52, 756.54, 756.55, 756.56, 756.59, 756.7, 756.71, 756.8, 756.83, 756.89, 756.9, 757.0, 758, 758.0, 758.3, 758.6, 758.7, 758.8, 758.81, 758.89, 758.9, 759.5, 759.59, 759.6, 759.7, 759.8, 759.81, 759.82, 759.83, 759.89

Cardiac and circulatory congenital anomalies: DX 745, 745.1, 745.6, 746, 746.0, 746.8, 747.1, 747.2

Digestive congenital anomalies: DX 751.6, 751.61

Genitourinary congenital anomalies: DX 752.7, 753.1, 753.10, 753.11, 753.15, 753.17, 753.2, 753.21, 753.22, 753.23

Hemolytic jaundice and perinatal jaundice: DX 774

Other perinatal conditions: DX 775.1, 775.2, 775.3

Joint disorders and dislocations, trauma-related: DX 717, 717.7, 717.8, 717.81, 717.82, 717.83, 717.84, 717.85, 717.89, 717.9, 718, 718.0, 718.00, 718.01, 718.02, 718.03, 718.04, 718.05, 718.07, 718.08, 718.09, 905.6

Fracture of upper limb: DX 905.2, 905.4

Other fractures: DX 905, 905.1, 905.5

Sprains and strains: DX 905.7

Intracranial injury: DX 907, 907.0

Open wounds of extremities: DX 905.8, 905.9

Conditions not to be used for assessing eligibility *(continued)*

Poisoning by other medications and drugs: DX 909, 909.0, 000.5

Poisoning by nonmedicinal substances: DX 909.1

Other injuries and conditions due to external causes: DX 907.1, 907.3, 907.4, 907.5, 907.9, 908.5, 908.6, 908.9, 909.2, 909.4, 909.9, 995.50, 995.51, 995.52, 995.80, 995.82, 995.84

Crushing injury or internal injury: DX 908

Gangrene: DX 440.24

Allergic reactions: DX 518.6

Rehabilitation care, fitting of prostheses, and adjustment of devices: DX V52

Residual codes, unclassified: DX 302, 302.0, 780.5, 780.50, 780.51, 780.52, 780.53, 780.54, 780.55, 780.56, 780.57, 780.59, V42.8, V42.81, V42.82, V42.83, V46, V46.0, V46.8, V46.9

References

Bennett, J. A., Perrin, N. A., Hanson, G., Bennett, D., Gaynor, W., Flaherty-Robb, M., et al. (2005). Healthy aging demonstration project: Nurse coaching for behavior change in older adults. *Research in Nursing and Health, 28*(3), 187–197.

Bodenheimer, T. (2003). Interventions to improve chronic illness care: Evaluating their effectiveness. *Disease Management, 6*(2), 63–71.

Bodenheimer, T. (2006). Primary care—Will it survive? *The New England Journal of Medicine, 355*(9), 861–864.

Bodenheimer, T., Wagner, E. H., & Grumbach, K. (2002). Improving primary care for patients with chronic illness. *Journal of the American Medical Association, 288*(14), 1775–1779.

Boult, C. (2006). The financing of health care for older people. In C. Christmas, S. R. Counsell, G. P. Eleazer, A. R. Fabiny, & S. K. Schultz (Eds.), *Geriatric Review Syllabus: A Core Curriculum in Geriatric Medicine* (6th ed.). New York: American Geriatrics Society.

Boult, C., Boult, L., Morishita, L., Dowd, B., Kane, R. L., & Urdangarin, C. (2001). A randomized trial of outpatient geriatric evaluation and management. *Journal of the American Geriatrics Society, 49*(4), 351–359.

Boult, C., Christmas, C., Durso, S. C., Leff, B., Boult, L., & Fried, L. P. (2008). Transforming chronic care for older persons. *Academic Medicine, 83*(3), 627–631.

Boult, C., Green, A., Boult, L., Pacala, J. T., Snyder, C., & Leff, B. (2008). *Successful models of comprehensive health care for multimorbid older persons: A review of effects on health and health care* (report to the Institute of Medicine). Washington, DC: National Academy of Sciences.

Boult, C., Reider, L., Frey, K., Leff, B., Boyd, C. M., Wolff, J. L., et al. (2008). The early effects of "Guided Care" on the quality of health care for multimorbid older persons: A cluster-randomized controlled trial. *Journals of Gerontology: Medical Sciences, 63(A)(3),* 321–327.

Boyd, C. M., Boult, C., Shadmi, E., Leff, B., Brager, R., Dunbar, L., et al. (2007). Guided Care for multimorbid older adults. *The Gerontologist, 47*(5), 697–704.

Boyd, C. M., Shadmi, E., Conwell, L. J., Griswold, M., Leff, B., Brager, R., et al. (2008). A pilot test of the effect of Guided Care on the quality of primary care experiences for multimorbid older adults. *Journal of General Internal Medicine, 23*(5), 536–542.

Callahan, C. M., Boustani, M. A., Unverzagt, F. W., Austrom, M. G., Damush, T. M., Perkins, A. J., et al. (2006). Effectiveness of collaborative care for older adults with Alzheimer's disease in primary care: A randomized controlled trial. *Journal of the American Medical Association, 295*(18), 2148–2157.

Campbell, S., Reeves, D., Kontopantelis, E., Middleton, E., Sibbald, B., & Roland, M. (2007). Quality of primary care in England with the introduction of pay for performance. *New England Journal of Medicine, 357*(2), 181–190.

Case Management Society of America. *2005 Case management salary survey results.* Retrieved July 31, 2008, from http://www.cmsa.org/portals/0/pdf/SalarySurvey2005.pdf

Centers for Medicare & Medicaid Services. (2008). *Medicare information on risk adjustment.* Retrieved July 31, 2008, from http://www.cms.hhs.gov/MedicareAdvtg SpecRateStats/06_Risk_adjustment.asp

Cohen, H. J., Feussner, J. R., Weinberger, M., Carnes, M., Hamdy, R. C., Hsieh, F., et al. (2002). A controlled trial of inpatient and outpatient geriatric evaluation and management. *New England Journal of Medicine, 346*(12), 905–912.

Coleman, E. A., Parry, C., Chalmers, S., & Min, S. J. (2006). The care transitions intervention: Results of a randomized controlled trial. *Archives of Internal Medicine, 166*(17), 1822–1828.

Counsell, S. R., Callahan, C. M., Clark, D. O., Tu, W., Buttar, A. B., Stump, T. E., et al. (2007). Geriatric care management for low-income seniors: A randomized controlled trial. *Journal of the American Medical Association, 298*(22), 2623–2633.

Darer, J. D., Hwang, W., Pham, H. H., Bass, E. B., & Anderson, G. (2004). More training needed in chronic care: A survey of U.S. physicians. *Academic Medicine, 79*(6), 541–548.

Davis, K., Schoen, C., Schoenbaum, S. C., Doty, M. M., Holmgren, A. L., Kriss, J. L., et al. (2007, May). *Mirror, mirror on the wall: An international update on the comparative performance of American health care, The Commonwealth Fund.* Retrieved July 31, 2008, from http://www.commonwealthfund.org/usr_doc/1027_Davis_mirror_ mirror_international_update_final.pdf?section=4039

Dorr, D. A., Wilcox, A. B., Brunker, C. P., Burdon, R. E., & Donnelly, S. M. (2008). The effect of technology-supported, multi-disease care management on the mortality and hospitalization of seniors. *Journal of the American Geriatric Society, 56*(12), 2203–2210.

Health Resources and Services Administration, Bureau of Health Professions. (2004). *The registered nurse population: 2004 national sample survey of registered nurses.* Retrieved July 31, 2008, from http://datawarehouse.hrsa.gov/nursingsurvey.htm

Holtz-Eakin, D. (2004). *An analysis of the literature on disease management programs.* Washington, DC: Congressional Budget Office.

Institute for Health Policy Solutions. (2005). *Risk adjustment methods and their relevance to "pay-or-play."* Retrieved July 31, 2008, from http://www.ihps.org/pubs/2005_Apr_ IHPS_SB2_ESup_Risk_Adj.pdf

Institute of Medicine. (1978). *Aging and medical education.* Washington, DC: National Academy of Sciences.

Institute of Medicine. (2001). *Crossing the quality chasm: A new health system for the 21st century.* Washington, DC: National Academy Press.

Institute of Medicine: Committee on Leadership for Academic Geriatric Medicine. (1987). Report of the Institute of Medicine: Academic geriatrics for the year 2000. *Journal of the American Geriatrics Society, 35,* 773–791.

Kane, R. L. (2002). The future history of geriatrics: Geriatrics at the crossroads. *Journals of Gerontology. Series A, Biological Sciences and Medical Sciences, 57*(12), M803–M805.

Leff, B., Reider, L., Frick, K., Scharfstein, D., Boyd, C., Frey, K., et al. (2009). "Guided Care" and the cost of complex health care. Manuscript in press.

Linden, A., & Adler-Milstein, J. (2008). Disease management program in policy context. *Health Care Financing Review, 29*(3), 1–11.

Lorig, K. R., & Holman, H. R. (2003). Self-management education: History, definition, outcomes, and mechanisms. *Annals of Behavioral Medicine, 26*(1), 1–7.

Lorig, K. R., Ritter, P., Stewart, A. L., Sobel, D. S., Brown, B. W., Jr., Bandura, A., et al. (2001). Chronic disease self-management program: Two-year health status and health care utilization outcomes. *Medical Care, 39*(11), 1217–1223.

Martin, J. C., Avant, R. F., Bowman, M. A., Bucholtz, J. R., Dickinson, J. R., Evans, K. L., et al. (2004). The future of family medicine: A collaborative project of the family medicine community. *Annals of Family Medicine, 2*(S1), S3–S32.

Naylor, M. D., Brooten, D., Campbell, R., Jacobsen, B. S., Mezey, M. D., Pauly, M. V., et al. (1999). Comprehensive discharge planning and home follow-up of hospitalized elders: A randomized clinical trial. *Journal of the American Medical Association, 281*(7), 613–620.

Neuman, P., Cubanski, J., Desmond, K. A., & Rice, T. H. (2007). How much 'skin in the game' do Medicare beneficiaries have? The increasing financial burden of health care spending, 1997–2003. *Health Affairs, 26*(6), 1692–1701.

Ofman, J. J., Badamgarav, E., Henning, J. M., Knight, K., Gano, A. D. J., Levan, R. K., et al. (2004). Does disease management improve clinical and economic outcomes in patients with chronic diseases? A systematic review. *The American Journal of Medicine, 117*(3), 182–192.

Pacala, J. T., Boult, C., Hepburn, K. W., Kane, R. A., Kane, R. L., Malone, J. K., et al. (1995). Case management of older adults in health maintenance organizations. *Journal of the American Geriatrics Society, 43*(5), 538–542.

Paulson, H. M., Chao, E. L., Leavitt, M. O., Astrue, M. J., & Weems, K. N. (2008). *Annual report of the board of trustees of the federal hospital insurance and federal supplementary Medicare insurance trust fund.* Retrieved July 31, 2008, from http://www.cms.hhs.gov/ReportsTrustFunds/downloads/tr2008.pdf

Phelan, E. A., Williams, B., Penninx, B. W., LoGerfo, J. P., & Leveille, S. G. (2004). Activities of daily living function and disability in older adults in a randomized trial of the health enhancement program. *Journals of Gerontology. Series A, Biological Sciences and Medical Sciences, 59*(8), 838–843.

Pope, G. C., Kautter, J., Ellis, R. P., Ash, A. S., Ayanian, J. Z., Lezzoni, L. I., et al. (2004). Risk adjustment of Medicare capitation payments using the CMS-HCC model. *Health Care Financing Review, 25*(4), 119–141.

Prochaska, J. O., & DiClemente, C. C. (1984). *The transtheoretical approach: Crossing traditional boundaries of therapy.* Homewood, IL: Dow Jones-Irwin.

Reuben, D. B., Frank, J. C., Hirsch, S. H., McGuigan, K. A., & Maly, R. C. (1999). A randomized clinical trial of outpatient comprehensive geriatric assessment coupled with an intervention to increase adherence to recommendations. *Journal of the American Geriatrics Society, 47*(3), 269–276.

Rollnick, S., Mason, P., & Butler, C. (1999). *Health Behavior Change: A Guide for Practitioners.* Edinburgh, Scotland: Churchill Livingstone.

Rowe, J. W., Allen-Meares, P. G., Altman, S. H., Bernard, M. A., Blumenthal, D., Chapman, S. A., et al. (2008). Preface in Buckwalter, K. C., Green Burger, S., Cassel, C. K., Dawson, S. L., Detmer, D., Ettinger, W. H., et al., *Retooling for an aging America: Building the health care workforce* (p. xii). Washington, DC: Institute of Medicine.

Rubin, C. D., Stieglitz, H., Vicioso, B., & Kirk, L. (2003). Development of geriatrics-oriented faculty in general internal medicine. *Annals of Internal Medicine, 139*(7), 615–620.

Salsberg, E., & Grover, A. (2006). Physician workforce shortages: Implications and issues for academic health centers and policymakers. *Academic Medicine, 81*(9), 782–787.

Sommers, L. S., Marton, K. I., Barbaccia, J. C., & Randolph, J. (2000). Physician, nurse, and social worker collaboration in primary care for chronically ill seniors. *Archives of Internal Medicine, 160*(12), 1825–1833.

Stuck, A. E., Egger, M., Hammer, A., Minder, C. E., & Beck, J. C. (2002). Home visits to prevent nursing home admission and functional decline in elderly people: Systematic review and meta-regression analysis. *Journal of the American Medical Association, 287*(8), 1022–1028.

Sylvia, M. L., Griswold, M., Dunbar, L., Boyd, C., Park, M., & Boult, C. (2008). Guided Care: Cost and utilization outcomes in a pilot study. *Disease Management, 11*(1), 29–36.

Unutzer, J., Katon, W., Callahan, C. M., Williams, J. W., Jr., Hunkeler, E., Harpole, L., et al. (2002). Collaborative care management of late-life depression in the primary care setting: A randomized controlled trial. *Journal of the American Medical Association, 288*(22), 2836–2845.

Warshaw, G. A., Bragg, E. J., Brewer, D. E., Meganathan, K., & Ho, M. (2007). The development of academic geriatric medicine: Progress toward preparing the nation's physicians to care for an aging population. *Journal of the American Geriatrics Society, 55*(12), 2075–2082.

Wenger, N. S., Solomon, D. H., Roth, C. P., MacLean, C. H., Saliba, D., Kamberg, C. J., et al. (2003). The quality of medical care provided to vulnerable community-dwelling older patients. *Annals of Internal Medicine, 139*(9), 740–747.

Wolff, J. L., Starfield, B., & Anderson, G. (2002). Prevalence, expenditures, and complications of multiple chronic conditions in the elderly. *Archives of Internal Medicine, 162*, 2269–2276.

Wolff, J. L., Rand-Giovanetti, E., Palmer, S., Wegener, S., Reider, L., Frey, K., et al. (in press). Caregiving and chronic care: The Guided Care program for families and friends. *Journals of Gerontology: Medical Sciences, 64*(A).

Index

ABIM. *See* American Board of Internal Medicine

Action Plans, 17, 18, 49, 94
  creation of, 92

Advertisements, 80

Alzheimer's Association, 21

Ambulatory care-sensitive conditions, 3

American Academy of Family Physicians, 69, 139, 149

American Board of Internal Medicine (ABIM), 139

American College of Physicians, 139, 149

American Geriatrics Society, 149

American Medical Group Association (AMGA), 140, 141

American Nurses Association (ANA), 90, 139, 146

American Nurses Credentialing Center, 73, 139, 146

AMGA. *See* American Medical Group Association

ANA. *See* American Nurses Association

Annual margin costs, 132

Applicant rating scale, 75

Application process, MMHD, 184–185

Area Agency on Aging, 18, 21, 61

Assessment
  caregiver, form, 109
  caregivers, 91
  patient, 91

Baby boomers, 1–2

Background information, 30–31

Baker, Ben, 5

Beneficiaries
  eligibility of, 136, 196–206
  MMHD, 192

Blood-related disease, 200

Board of Nursing, 146

Budgets, 131–141

Bush, George W., 182

Calls to patient, 90

Cancer, 198–199

Caregivers
  assessment form, 109
  assessment of, 91
  educating and supporting, 20
  invitation letter, 108
  preparing, 70–71
  support, 121